"So many of the people who write me at 'Savage Love' are curious about kink—some days it accounts for half the mail—but they don't know where to start. I'm going to be recommending this collection of essays. This is more than just a guide to kink, it's more than a sex manual. Editor Tristan Taormino has brought the players, thinkers, and rock stars of the kink scene and together they have created a book that not only lets people know where to start, but why to start, and what they'll get out of it. Vanillas, novices, old hands, old guard—everyone can learn from this collection."

—Dan Savage

"Tristan Taormino has gifted us with a magnificent collection of essays from kinkdom's finest educators: consider it required reading for every kinkster who lives life on the hot side."

—Dossie Easton, co-author of
The New Topping Book and *The New Bottoming Book*

"Tristan Taormino has created a perfect compendium of kink that covers the nuts and bolts of spanking, bondage, role playing, rough sex, and much more, as well as the philosophies, motivations, and deeply personal experiences of an array of BDSM players. If 'Brutal Affection' sounds like an oxymoron to you, read on. Keep a copy in your bedroom—and your toy bag!"

—Rachel Kramer Bussel,
editor of *Spanked* and *Best Sex Writing 2012*

"Finally, a smart, comprehensive, and brave book on kinky sex for this generation. Tristan Taormino's *The Ultimate Guide to Kink* is the first really good new book on the subject in years. BDSM and kink aficionados are lifelong learners, endlessly fascinated with their own sexual and personal growth. I expect this to be the BDSM bible for the next decade."

—Felice Newman,
author of *The Whole Lesbian Sex Book*

The Ultimate Guide
to Kink

The Ultimate Guide to Kink:

BDSM, Role Play and the Erotic Edge

**EDITED BY
TRISTAN TAORMINO**

Copyright © 2012 by Tristan Taormino.
Illustrations copyright @ 2012 by Katie Diamond

All rights reserved. Except for brief passages quoted in newspaper, magazine, radio, television, or online reviews, no part of this book may be reproduced in any form or by any means, electronic or mechanical, including photocopying or recording, or by information storage or retrieval system, without permission in writing from the publisher.

Published in the United States by Cleis Press, Inc.,
221 River Street, 9th Floor, Hoboken, NJ 07030

Cover design: Scott Idleman/Blink
Cover photograph, top left: Michael Hitoshi/Getty Images
Cover photograph, top right: Christine Kessler
Cover photograph, bottom left: WIN-Initiative
Cover photograph, bottom right: John Ross/Getty Images
Text design: Frank Wiedemann

Trade paper ISBN: 978-1-57344-779-9
E-book ISBN: 978-1-57344-782-9

Library of Congress Cataloging-in-Publication Data

The ultimate guide to kink : BDSM, role play, and the erotic edge / edited by Tristan Taormino.
p. cm.
ISBN 978-1-57344-779-9 (pbk.)
1. Bondage (Sexual behavior) 2. Sadomasochism. I. Taormino, Tristan, 1971-

HQ79.U485 2012
306.77'5--dc23

2011049976

CONTENTS

Introduction: Playing on the Erotic Edge
    Tristan Taormino xi

Part 1 *Skills and Techniques* 1

1. "S is for...": The Terms, Principles, and Pleasures of Kink
    Tristan Taormino. 3
2. Making an Impact: Spanking, Caning, and Flogging
    Lolita Wolf 33
3. How to Train Your Sex Slave
    Laura Antoniou 54
4. Whole Hand Sex: Vaginal Fisting and BDSM
    Sarah Sloane 69
5. Bondage for Sex
    Midori 87
6. A Little Cock and Ball Play
    Hardy Haberman 125
7. Kinky Twisted Tantra
    Barbara Carrellas 139
8. Piercing Scenes
    FifthAngel 169
9. Brutal Affection: Playing with Rough Sex
    Felice Shays 186
10. Butthole Bliss: The Ins and Outs of Anal Fisting
    Patrick Califia 224

Part 2 *Fantasies and Philosophies* 245

11. Stop, Drop, and Role! Erotic Role Playing
    Mollena Williams 247

12. A Romp on the Wild Side: Erotic Human Animal Role Playing
    Lee Harrington 264

13. ForteFemme: The Art and Philosophy of Feminine Dominance
    Midori... 280

14. Submissive: A Personal Manifesto
    Madison Young 297

15. Enhancing Masochism: How to Expand Limits and Increase Desire
    Patrick Califia 309

16. Inside the Mind of a Sadist
    FifthAngel 333

17. Age Role Play
    Ignacio Rivera, aka Papí Coxxx 352

18. Digging in the Dirt: The Lure of Taboo Role Play
    Mollena Williams 366

19. The Dark Side
    Jack Rinella.................................... 388

20. Mindfuck
    Edge 404

Resource Guide...................................... 429
About the Contributors 436
About the Illustrator 447
About the Editor 448

ILLUSTRATIONS

Chapter 4

    71   Plate 4.1. Female anatomy

Chapter 5

    94   Plate 5.1. Simple scarf wrist tie

    96   Plate 5.2. Midori's dildo harness

    98   Plate 5.3. Scarf sex sling

    104   Plate 5.4. Simple single-column rope tie

    106   Plate 5.5. Simple double-column rope tie

    108   Plate 5.6. Open-leg crab variation

    110   Plate 5.7. Rope sex sling

    113   Plate 5.8. Japanese bondage

Chapter 7

    153   Plate 7.1. Simple rope handcuffs

    158   Plate 7.2. Yab Yum

    160   Plate 7.3. Heart energy exchange

Chapter 8

    174   Plate 8.1. Piercing needles

    177   Plate 8.2. Needle insertion

Chapter 9

    210   Plate 9.1. Where to strike

INTRODUCTION: PLAYING ON THE EROTIC EDGE

This book is for everyone who dares to expand their erotic horizons beyond the ordinary. For all those who like to give and receive intense sensations. For the people who eroticize power and cultivate consciousness in sex and relationships. For anyone who loves to dance on the line between pleasure and pain. For folks who nurture naked creativity and make fantasies come to life. This book is about kink.

Kink is an intimate experience, an exchange of power between people that can be physical, erotic, sexual, psychological, spiritual, or, most often, some combination. I use the word *kink* as an all-encompassing term to describe the people, practices, and communities that move beyond traditional ideas about sex to explore the edges of eroticism. Kink is meant to include BDSM, sadomasochism, kinky sex, dominance and submission, role play, sex games, fantasy, fetish, and other alternative erotic expressions.

Whatever you call it, the popularity of kink has soared in the last 25 years. The Internet has changed the landscape dramatically, and it's no surprise that kinky folk were early adopters of electronic bulletin boards and Listservs. Today, we have access to information, resources, and other like-minded people as never before. What used to be a covert world with its own symbols, traditions, and underground gatherings, where people were afraid to use their real names, has become a visible, accessible subculture. When someone expresses an interest in kink, I always give the same advice: find your local community. Want to know where the kinksters are in your neighborhood? Google BDSM and your town, city, or county, and you'll come up with social events, workshops, support groups, conferences, and, for lucky folks, play parties, dungeons, and clubs.

There are hundreds of gatherings of kinksters throughout North America—whether it's a local organization's annual conference, a camping event for pervy people, or a BDSM retreat—and the majority of them have a strong educational component. On any given weekend, you can learn how to: safely set someone on fire, be a good Daddy, plan the perfect gang bang, do bondage without rope, or channel your inner shaman. As a group, people into kink devote a lot of time, resources, and energy to learning.

I first heard the phrase *lifelong learners* when a friend of mine who works at a public radio station told me that marketers use it to refer to NPR listeners.[1] Lifelong learners are people who are self-motivated to continually seek out new knowledge and skills, through informal and formal education, to constantly develop and improve themselves.[2] The concept really resonates with me, as it aptly describes so many of the people I meet at sex and kink events—we are lifelong learners. That's what's so ironic about the conservative backlash against BDSMers. With increased visibility comes increased bigotry, and conservatives continue to rally against kinky events by local groups to get them shut down. What the anti-kink fanatics don't understand about us is that we're geeks. Sex nerds. SM intellectuals. We pay money to spend a weekend going to *classes*.

Of course, we do manage to get our noses out of the books to have fun, too. In the process of having a good time and getting off, we also strive to create alternative utopian worlds, even if only for a weekend. The kink community is built on the radical notion that people can express their erotic needs and desires and have them met. We believe that dreams do come true, and not at Disneyland, but in our bedrooms. Kink events are not just about getting together to have fabulous erotic experiences. We learn skills that we can translate into every part of our life: how to claim our desires, negotiate for what we want and need, set boundaries, communicate limits, acknowledge power dynamics, celebrate sexuality, and accept each other's differences.

I envisioned this book as a compilation of the work of some of the best educators in North America, and every piece was written specifically for it. You don't have to attend dozens of regional or national events to hear these experts speak—they are gathered here, in one place, taking on topics about which they are truly passionate. Their expertise in these subjects is tremendous, yet some of them have never had their writing about kink published for a wide audience. As you turn the pages, I want you to feel as if you're at one of these gatherings, spending time with the teachers as they share their wisdom, experience, thoughts, opinions, and personal anecdotes. Unlike books about BDSM only, the chapters in this book explore different areas of kink with a specific focus on sex. After all, sex is a big part of what motivates and manifests our kink, but, until recently, it was often left out of the equation in our educational offerings.

The book is divided into two sections. In "Skills and Techniques," pieces feature nuts-and-bolts, how-to tutorials, sprinkled with lots of creative ideas and examples. You'll learn about topics from bondage and spanking to piercing and rough sex. This section is beautifully illustrated by queer artist Katie Diamond, who created the images expressly for this book. There are a variety of role-playing fantasies as well as personal manifestos in the second section, "Fantasies and Philosophies." From masochism to age play, these pieces cover some of the edgiest and most taboo and controversial elements of kink in depth. The subjects, which have long been a part of kink, are too rarely discussed outside closed circles or in print. It's time to shine a light on what is often only perceived as darkness.

I wanted the collection to capture not only the incredible exchange of ideas at kink conferences, but the magic that happens at a gathering of a kinky tribe. I hope you learn a lot from this diverse group of writers and you are inspired to find them, and other educators, at an event near you so you can supplement this education with mentoring, hands-on demonstrations, and interactive learning.

Exploring kink provides us with an opportunity for self-reflection, challenge, and personal growth. Where many people are content to just sit back and let life happen, we're not: we constantly engage our identities, sexualities, and relationships. Sometimes, it's about testing ourselves. Rock climbing aficionados, competitive triathletes, or ambitious innovators in the business world: there are those who strive to go farther, faster, deeper. Some of us don't do it dangling from a mountain; we do it through intense—what some would call extreme—erotic experiences. Kink can be a private (or semi-public) laboratory—a sacred space where we feel safe enough to try new things, push our boundaries, flirt with edges, and conquer fears. Because it combines the physical, emotional, psychological, and spiritual, it has the potential to heal old wounds and generate spiritual renewal. It can deepen our connections and relationships, bringing a new level of intimacy to them. Kink is a crucible for creativity, vulnerability, perseverance, control, catharsis, and connection. Kink is a unique space where there is room to experiment and see what bubbles up.

Tristan Taormino
New York

Endnotes

1. Some elements of this introduction, including the concept of kinky people as lifelong learners, are adapted from my 2009 keynote talk for Winter Wickedness in Columbus, Ohio. My thanks to Barak and Brat Sheba of Adventures in Sexuality for inviting me to give that talk.

2. The roots of the phrase are in the concept of lifelong learning, defined in a statement by the European Lifelong Learning Initiative and the American Council on Education: "Lifelong learning is the development of human potential through a continuously supportive process which stimulates and empowers individuals to acquire all the knowledge, values, skills, and understanding they will require throughout their lifetimes and to apply them with confidence, creativity and enjoyment in all roles, circumstances, and environments." Norman Longworth and Keith W. Davies, *Lifelong Learning: New Vision, New Implications, New Roles for People, Organizations, Nations and Communities in the 21st Century* (London: Kogan Page, 1996), 22.

Skills and Techniques

CHAPTER 1

"S IS FOR...": THE TERMS, PRINCIPLES, AND PLEASURES OF KINK

TRISTAN TAORMINO

Like other subcultures, kinky folks have developed (and continue to develop) a vocabulary to describe the unique elements of our world. This chapter will define the most common words and phrases used among kink practitioners and throughout the book.

In addition to a specific vernacular, members of the kink community have adopted a set of principles that represent its core values: consent, negotiation, safety and risk reduction, communication, and aftercare. These values are the foundation of the work of all the educators in this book, and they apply to each of the chapters and all of the activities discussed here. To avoid repetition, most authors will not define basic terms or tenets covered here, although they may elaborate on them or define other terminology as it relates specifically to their topic.

TERMINOLOGY AND LINGO
Kink
In this book, *kink* is used as an inclusive term that covers BDSM, sadomasochism, kinky sex, dominance and submission, role play, sex games, fantasy, fetish, and other alternative erotic expressions.

BDSM
BDSM is an acronym and an umbrella term that was first used in the late 80s and early 90s in Internet discussion groups, including one of the early newsgroups, soc.subculture.bondage-bdsm. It did not become the umbrella term of choice until the 2000s. *BDSM* is a combination of several shorter acronyms that reflect the history of our kinky vocabulary and the wide variety of practices that it incorporates:

B & D or *B/D* stands for bondage and discipline. It is an older term that first appeared in personals and magazines in the 1970s and became widely used by kinky folks in the 1980s to describe their interest in kink. It wasn't necessarily meant to denote *only* bondage and discipline, but rather a range of activities that revolved around power exchange. Today *B & D* is much less frequently used as a term on its own.

SM (also *S & M*, *S/M*, *S/m*) is the common abbreviation for sadism and masochism or sadomasochism. (Definitions of these and related words appear later in this chapter.) These terms were coined by Richard von Krafft-Ebing in 1886 and have appeared frequently since then in psychoanalytic literature to describe sexual pathologies; however, kinky people reclaimed them beginning around the 1970s, and *S/M* was the most popular term until *BDSM* gained widespread use by the 2000s.

Embedded in the acronym *BDSM* is *D/s* (also *DS* or *d/s*), which represents dominance and submission or Dominant/submissive (defined in detail below). These terms have been around for a long time; people began using them in the context of kink in the 1980s to describe the power dynamic within a scene or relationship. People used *D/s* to reflect the power exchange in SM activities or to communicate their interest in roles like master/slave or daddy/boy, for example. Today, *D/s* is most often used to denote relationships that are built around a dominant/submissive power dynamic where power exchange is always or very often present (and may exist without other elements of BDSM).[1] In those D/s relationships where the power exchange is always present, partners inhabit their roles and reinforce the dynamic through various rituals, protocols, and behaviors all the time; these relationships may be referred to as *24/7 D/s* (as in 24 hours a day, 7 days a week), *lifestyle D/s*, *TPE* (total power exchange), or *APE* (absolute power exchange).

BDSM can be used as a noun ("I'm interested in BDSM") or an adjective ("I went to a BDSM event"). Some people use other terms interchangeably with BDSM, including SM, kink, and leather. The use of the word *leather* (as in "I'm part of the local leather community") originated in post-World War II gay male biker clubs and bars and continued in leather bars and sex clubs from the late 50s all the way through the 2000s.² *Leather* is still used today, especially by gay, lesbian, bisexual, transgender, and queer folks, to signify kinky interests, identities, and communities.

People do BDSM for the same wide variety of reasons people have sex, including for pleasure and connection. Just as some people love oral sex and others love sex in the woods, some love BDSM. Plenty of folks have told me they believe it's just how they're wired. I've heard countless stories of the first time a lover held her down, the first time a woman put a collar on him, the first time she got spanked. Many experienced a visceral reaction to these experiences before they had language to describe what they were doing or knew there were other people out there doing similar things. For some, BDSM does not have to focus on or even involve genital stimulation to be pleasurable and even orgasmic. For others, a good flogging and a good fucking is the perfect combination—BDSM enhances the sexual experience.

In sidebars throughout this chapter, you'll find examples of different kinds of BDSM as well as popular practices and tools. I hope they illustrate the extraordinary diversity within BDSM, provide you with a list of possibilities, and whet your appetite for the chapters to come.³

Play is a common term used to describe the practice of BDSM, as in: "I want to play with a bondage expert so I can learn more about it." It can also be used as an adjective: "My play partner caned me really well at Susan's play party. I'm glad I set up that play date!"

A *scene* is where two or more people come together

to do BDSM. People may also use *scene* to describe the BDSM community ("Is she in the scene?"). You can do a scene anywhere, but often people do them in a play space or dungeon. These spaces may be private, such as a room in someone's home, or public, like a large club; they often have different stations that feature various types of equipment for BDSM play: for example, a St. Andrew's Cross (a large X usually made of wood), a bondage bed, a spanking bench, a sling, a medical exam table, and a cage.

> ## WHACK!
>
> *When I feel the pounding of a heavy flogger (or anything with a heavy thud) against my ass or thighs, I feel this amazing connection to life and to my partner. I also feel this huge thick chunk of energy making contact with my body and then dissipating from that point of contact throughout the rest of my body.*
>
> —MADISON
>
> **Impact play:** spanking, caning, slapping, flogging, Florentine flogging, and whipping
>
> **Tools:** hands, paddles, canes, slappers, crops, floggers, quirts, singletail whips

EXPLORE DIFFERENT SENSATIONS

I stood over her as she lay on the massage table. I stared intently into her eyes. I pinched a section of flesh of her inner thigh, pressed firmly, then tugged a little. She squirmed, so I pinched harder. She gasped, then giggled. One by one, I put bright red plastic clothespins in a line until she had a dozen, six on each side. Then I pulled out a special pair: shiny silver magnetic clothespins. My mom put them in my stocking for Christmas. "Won't those be useful?" she said, imagining me clipping important documents to the filing cabinet in my office. "Oh, yes they will," I smirked. I saved them for a very sensitive spot: right where the leg meets the crotch, an inch away from her wet pussy.

After the initial pain when a clip first goes on, the circulation stops and you just feel pressure. I could tell she was proud of herself, probably thinking, This isn't so bad. She had no idea what was in store for her when the clips came off: a searing pain that can be pleasurable for some, almost intolerable for others, and intense no matter what. I tugged at the first one, squeezed the end, and released her skin. She breathed in sharply, then exhaled deeply.

Sensation play: clips and clamps, pinching, hot wax, knife play (without breaking the skin), electricity play, tickle torture, cupping, fire cupping, fire play

Tools: nipple clamps, clothespins, zippers (clothespins or clips strung together) clips, candles, vampire gloves, knives, TENS unit, violet wand, cups

Tops, Bottoms, and Switches

During a scene, a *top* is the "doer," the person who is in charge, initiates activities and actions, and does things to the bottom. A *bottom* follows the top's lead, receives stimulation from the top, and has things done to him or her. For example, in a spanking scene, the top is the spanker and the bottom gets spanked. Top and bottom can also be used as verbs, as in "I topped my girlfriend last night." A switch is someone who enjoys playing both roles. Whether a switch becomes a top or a bottom can change from one scene to the next; switches may take on a particular role based on the partner they play with or the activity. They can also switch between both roles within one scene.

Sadomasochism

Sadomasochism is the enjoyment of giving or receiving pain or discomfort. A *sadist* is one who derives pleasure from inflicting pain, intense sensations, and discomfort on someone else. That pain or discomfort can be physical (like during a spanking), emotional and psychological (as in an interrogation scene), or both. This is just a brief definition; Chapter 16, Inside the Mind of a Sadist, by FifthAngel, is a thorough, thoughtful look at sadism. A *masochist* is someone who enjoys receiving pain or intense sensations, being made uncomfortable, or being "forced" to do something they don't enjoy. Remember that sadists and masochists experience these desires and pleasures in the context of consensual BDSM scenes.

GET ROUGH

I enjoy being restrained but my preference is to be held down by human force; I like the feeling of hands squeezing my wrists and a knee on my chest, a hard palm pushing on my face. I also enjoy being called names and told that I am only good for fucking and for giving the other person pleasure. Something about being used makes me feel really hot and confident and empowered. Feeling out of control when there is trust and desire involved takes me to a transcendent place that I don't get to on my own or during non-BDSM sex.

—DYLAN

Rough body play: slapping, face slapping, hair pulling, spitting, punching, pushing, wrestling, biting, scratching

Tools: hands, mouths, bodies, boxing and other gloves

Let's talk about pain, since it's part of SM and comes to mind when people think of activities like flogging, caning, or piercing. When people experience pain, adrenaline, endorphins, and natural painkillers flood their nervous system. People get off on this chemical rush, which many describe as feeling energized, high, or transcendent. Pain is not just a physical event; like many things in our culture, it is also socially constructed and reinforced. When we see a person slap someone's face, we think, That hurt, that was unpleasant. But, in the context of a sexually charged scene, some people, when they are aroused (and their pain tolerance is much higher), process a face slap in a different way: it feels *good*. They like how their flesh responds and their pulse quickens. It may feel shocking, intimate, stinging; add the taboo of dominance, punishment, humiliation—whatever that slap signifies for the two people—and you've got a recipe for an intense experience. In certain contexts, one person's pain can be another person's pleasure. Or, as Patrick Califia writes in Chapter 15, Enhancing Masochism: How to Expand Limits and Increase Desire, which delves much deeper into this subject, "Euphoria and agony are next-door neighbors."

Dominance and Submission

A *Dominant* runs the show, exerts control over a submissive, and may direct him or her to complete tasks, behave a certain way, follow rules, or submit to various kinds of SM. A *submissive* gives up control and surrenders to the Dominant, complies with a Dominant's wishes, follows orders, and has an investment in pleasing his or her Dominant.

A power exchange of some kind is nearly always present in human relationships. There are people all around us in power exchange relationships who don't acknowledge the dynamic or call it anything: A husband who gives his wife an allowance but no credit card in her own name. A woman who controls her coworkers, making them eager to please her even though she's not their boss. That's right: there are plenty of people wearing collars and others tugging at their leashes, but the gear is invisible and the dynamic unexamined. Kinky people do the opposite: they consciously *create and name* a power dynamic in order to eroticize it. By making the power exchange explicit, they get to act on it, play with it, and let it drive the erotic interaction. That exchange is what fuels their desire and pleasure. Think about the mistress who forces her slave to be sexually available to her at all times. Or the submissive who strives to please her Dominant, putting his needs above her own.

Service is one kind of D/s dynamic or relationship where the submissive serves the Dominant; the Dominant may direct the submissive to do household chores, provide sexual stimulation, or complete projects. In fact, ordinary activities that most people take for granted—making coffee, drawing a bath, folding laundry—can be imbued with a different meaning and become symbols of submission and service. Service is most often equated with submissives (slaves, boys, girls, etc.), but there are also self-identified *service tops*, who enjoy doing things to bottoms at the bottom's request.

D/s roles and relationships are explored throughout the book, most extensively by Laura Antoniou (Chapter 3), Midori (Chapter 13), and Madison Young (Chapter 14).

Some people take on the role of Dominant or submissive expressly for a scene, like top or bottom, and shed that role when the scene ends. For others, being dominant or submissive is not about role playing, but is a much bigger part of their identity and relationships. For example, some Dominants can't turn their desire to dominate on and off at will, and they describe dominance as very similar to how people define sexual orientation: they are attracted to and interested in submissives, they

> ### PLAY WITH YOUR BITS
>
> *It gets me off better than anything else. You just can't be any fuller than when you have someone's entire hand inside you. It's emotional, even spiritual for me. It's the only act that can actually move me to tears, but they are good tears.*
>
> —CHLOE
>
> **Genitals, sex, and bodily fluids:** vaginal fisting, anal fisting, rough sex, cock and ball play, genital play and genitorture, sounds, enemas, watersports/golden showers
>
> **Tools:** hands, clips and clamps, menthol rub, rope, cock rings, gloves, lube, sex toys, needles

see the world through their dominant lens, their dominance is a constant in their sexual and BDSM interactions.

Many tops are dominant—their needs and wishes come first—and many bottoms are submissive—their desire is to please and serve their top. However, that is not always the case. For example, if a dominant master orders his submissive to flog him, then the master is the flogging bottom and the submissive is the flogging top; the master is still the one in charge, he's just having something done to him. The roles of sadist and masochist overlap with the others and many people identify with different elements of more than one. Sometimes the overlap is easily recognized, like a submissive masochist bottom who enjoys being flogged to experience both the pain and the submission to his Dominant's flogger. But there could also be a sadistic submissive who enjoys piercing masochist bottoms.

EROTIC ROLE PLAY

When you engage in erotic role play (also called fantasy role play), you and a partner (or partners) create characters and scenarios to act out fantasies with a sexual component. Erotic role play is a chance to become someone else, channel your inner drama geek, explore a particular dynamic, and have some fun. For some people, role play is part of their BDSM. It makes sense: most of the common role play scenarios—doctor/patient, teacher/student, cop/civilian, prostitute/client—have a power dynamic built right into them, and so much of BDSM is about power. Often these scenes revolve around one person submitting to another, being forced to do something, or feeling vulnerable. Think of a naughty student spanked by a ruler-wielding nun, a dominatrix humiliating her client, or a drill sergeant putting a private through his paces.

Other people may love erotic role play—and their scenarios can include corporal punishment, bondage, or mindfuck—but they don't consider what they do BDSM. There is plenty of overlap between erotic role play and BDSM: roles, scenarios, props, power dynamics, and, of course, getting off on all of it! It's entirely up to you. Many of the same principles adopted by BDSMers are also practiced by erotic role players and vice versa, which is why there are several chapters in this book

> ## IN THE DARK
>
> *I'm blindfolded and gagged on a pillow in a cold basement. I can feel the cool air and hear water dripping. I hear high heels coming closer and I'm struck across my ass and chest, slowly increasing in intensity. She straddles my shoulders after a good flogging and orders me to pleasure her. Right before she is about to come, she moves away and finishes herself off while all I can do is listen to her moans and screams.*
>
> —CHASE
>
> **Sensory deprivation:** sight deprivation, sound deprivation, scent deprivation, gagging, mummification, breath control and play
>
> **Tools:** blindfolds, hoods, earplugs, nose plugs, ball gags, mouth bits

about role play.

Fantasy role play gives folks a chance to be someone else, even if it's only for an hour or two. You can shake off your real-life stern, responsible school principal and become a pampered princess with a doting babysitter. Role play creates a space for fantasy and make-believe, where you can explore your inner cocky jock, naughty schoolgirl, or bored-but-horny housewife. It can add another layer to your sex life, where you explore the many facets of your own personality, different dynamics with a partner, sexual taboos, and scenarios limited only by your imagination.

PRINCIPLES

Consent

Consent—explicit, informed verbal approval after negotiation, a confident and secure "Yes!"—is the bedrock of sex and relationships, and one of the most significant elements of kink. It's what separates kink from abuse. It is something you will read about repeatedly in this book. Securing consent from a partner is a necessity, and this holds true whether the person is brand-new to you, you've played together more than a dozen times, or you've been in a relationship for 10 years. Never assume anything. When you ask for consent, you clearly speak your part in the exchange: I need to know you've agreed to this before we begin. Giving your consent to a partner prior to a scene is absolutely critical. It establishes that you're ready, willing, and able to proceed: you've discussed what's likely to happen, shared any concerns, talked about your limits, and agreed to dive in. When you give consent, you do so willingly, without pressure, coercion, or reservation. You agree to play, communicate during the scene, and stop if you need to.

Negotiation

Giving your consent and receiving a partner's consent is part of the process of negotiating a kink scene. Negotiation creates a space for everyone to talk about their needs, wants, limits, fantasies, and fears before they play. One way to begin the negotiation process is to identify what role or roles you will take on: top/bottom/switch, Dominant/submissive, sadist/masochist. Together you can go through some possible activities; for each one, you can decide if you are interested in doing it and whether you want to give or receive or both.

People sometimes make a "Yes–No–Maybe" list, marking "yes" for the things they'd like to do, "no" for the things they definitely wouldn't like to do, and "maybe" for activities that fall in between. A "maybe" can have multiple meanings; for example: maybe since I am curious but have no idea if I'll like it; maybe after I've had more experience with some other things; maybe if we get to know each other better and it feels right; maybe if I learn to get over my anxiety about it; or maybe because it's not a definitive "no," I'm open to the idea. It will serve you well to discuss why something ends up in the "maybe" column and will give you insight into your partner. The activities listed in the sidebars are a good place to start the conversation.

In addition to negotiating your wants, needs, desires, and limits for BDSM, you should also decide if there will be sexual activity as part of your play. You can write up a similar "Yes–No–Maybe" list. Will there be genital contact and stimulation? Masturbation? How about penetration, oral sex, sex toys, ejaculation? As part of the negotiation process, you should disclose when you were last tested for sexually transmitted infections (STIs) and decide on safer sex practices. (See UltimateGuidetoKink.com for a sample Yes–No–Maybe list and an STI/safer sex guide.)

Making a list of activities is like drawing the outline. Now it's time to fill in the details and get more specific. Erotic desire is in the details, so it's helpful to you and your partners to flesh out your fantasies and figure out exactly what you want. Say you like the idea of bondage. Do you crave being restrained into submission or do you like the idea of struggling to get out of it? You enjoy dominating. Do you prefer to give orders, create predicaments, or use someone for your pleasure? You know you're into sex-for-money fantasies where you're a prostitute—but are you a streetwalking hustler or a high-priced call girl?

THE ART OF RESTRAINT

As I stand there and each piece of rope gets laid across me, my focus changes. I get calmer and breathe deeper, and I can feel each fiber of the rope against my skin. With each layer, he controls more of my body. I bend as he wants me to, my flesh manipulated by his hands and the rope. It is no longer about voluntary compliance. As he taps my inner thigh to indicate I should move it, I hesitate. I know the moment I do move, he will know just how turned on I am from the scent between my legs permeating the air around us.

—KAITE

Bondage: rope bondage, cuffs, metal bondage, Japanese bondage, suspension, chastity devices, predicament bondage, mummification, confinement

Tools: rope, belts, ties, leather restraints, metal cuffs, bondage mitts, chastity belts, collars, leashes, athletic tape and wraps, bondage tape, plastic wrap, arm binders, sleep sacks, body bags, spreader bars, straitjackets, cages

As you fill in the details of your desires, decide on and communicate your limits within a certain activity; for example:

- *You love to be slapped and spanked, but not on your face.*
- *You're excited to have hot wax dripped on you, but you don't want it on your breasts.*
- *You checked "yes" under clips and clamps although you have one caveat: no clothespins.*
- *You're game to try sensory deprivation if your partner promises not to put a gag in your mouth.*
- *Caning is fun, but no marks on your body that people could see when you wear shorts.*

Now is also the time to tell your partner all relevant information he or she should know about you. Is there anything in your medical history that is serious or will affect the type of play you do? For example, you should let a partner know if you have a heart condition, high blood pressure, diabetes, or allergies. You should talk about medications you take, a sensitivity to hot or cold, if you're prone to dizziness or fainting, how well you can see without your glasses. Do you have bad knees and can't kneel for more than 20 minutes? That's vital information to tell a Dominant before a scene!

Although it can be difficult, you should also share any specific elements that you know can trigger a negative reaction in you; these may be based on phobias, negative experiences, past trauma, childhood abuse, or strong aversions.

They can be about a specific body part, an activity, an implement, a certain word or words. For example, I have a friend who cannot be spanked with a hairbrush because she has awful memories of being punished as a little girl with a hairbrush by her mother. Another friend likes to be called names like *whore* or *bitch* in a scene, but draws the line at *cow* or *pig*. I know a guy who has an intense fear of being strangled, so even hands around his neck can send him into a tailspin. A woman had a bad first-time experience with nipple clamps and now they give her tremendous anxiety.

This is important information to know as you decide if you're going to play with someone, what you're going to do, and how to construct a scene. This information sharing is part of giving and receiving *informed* consent; it also helps prepare you to assess the risks and determine how to play safer.

Safety, Risk, and Responsibility
The issues of safety and responsibility have been vital for kinky people both personally and politically. People who practice BDSM have long emphasized the importance of mentoring and education so newcomers can learn proper skills before picking up a paddle or a piercing needle. When SM groups first became more visible, and as they continue to grow and get more politically active, kinksters want nonkinky folks to know that they aren't whip-toting lunatics.

In 1983, the phrase "safe, sane, and consensual" (abbreviated *SSC*) appeared in a committee report of Gay Male S/M Activists (GMSMA) in New York; it is widely credited to David Stein, a member of GMSMA.[4] The concept of SSC was promoted to accomplish two goals: to articulate the values of a growing community and, as the practice of SM became increasingly visible, to raise awareness among the larger gay community that SM was not the same thing as abuse. Other SM communities and players embraced Stein's phrase with

> ## POWER EXCHANGE
>
> *I think I have the classic "businessman syndrome," where being in control all the time and having to make decisions all the time makes you crave someone else's control and want to submit. For me it is very freeing to know that my only obligation is to please someone else. Usually I am the one in charge of everything. It's great to have someone doing that for me.*
>
> —DONNA
>
> **Scene or relationship dynamics:** master/slave, domestic servitude, sexual service, personal service, 24/7 D/s

gusto as a kind of motto, and it quickly became a much-used catchphrase.

A decade after it was so widely embraced, some people began to interpret, critique, and debate the concept of SSC; they questioned whether it sanitized SM and was used to shame people who did more "risky" activities. Sex educators encourage people to practice safer sex, by using barriers, testing regularly, and developing other strategies to reduce the transmission of sexually transmitted infections (STIs). Educators emphasize that it's *safer* sex—not safe sex—to make the point that all sex comes with some risks. Likewise, critics of SSC wanted to acknowledge that one can take steps to be safer, but there is some kind of risk in all forms of BDSM.

In 1999, a new phrase was introduced: "risk-aware consensual kink" (RACK).[5] RACK continues to emphasize the consensual nature of BDSM while acknowledging that some of its practices are inherently risky (and, in fact, exploring the risks and edges are part of what draws people to them). You can make an informed decision to acknowledge the risks, take steps to reduce them, and proceed. Stein himself later clarified the context and intentions behind the creation of SSC and acknowledged some of its limitations:

> What we meant by "safe S/M" back in 1983—as the full GMSMA statement of purpose implies—was the opposite of careless, irresponsible, or uninformed S/M. We meant doing your homework and taking reasonable precautions. We never intended to promote only G-rated S/M or to turn the leather scene into a risk-free playpen where pain doesn't really hurt, bondage isn't really constraining, and dominance is being ordered to do what you want to do anyway.[6]

One way to reduce risk is to use a *safeword*. Although you negotiate and discuss limits, boundaries, and triggers before a scene, you cannot prepare for everything. It's simply impossible to predict how you'll feel during a scene, what will push your buttons, or how something will affect you.

A safeword is a word—usually one that you wouldn't normally utter during a scene—that you and your partner choose. Your safeword is your safety net. If you don't like something that's happening and you want the scene to stop right away, simply say your safeword. Words like *stop* or *no* or *please don't*, which we commonly use to communicate this sentiment, may be part of the dialogue of a scene where the bottom wants to resist or be forced to do something. So they are not ideal safewords. The most common safeword is *red*. Sometimes people pick two different words; for example, red means "stop right now!" and yellow means "please slow down." If the bottom can't speak (he has a gag in his mouth or she is supposed to perform oral sex until you tell her to stop) or the music is really loud in the dungeon, agree on a safe signal instead. For instance, you can have the bottom hold something in her hand during a scene; if she drops it, that means stop.

Another way to reduce risk is to know what you're doing. Luckily, there is a tremendous emphasis on education in the BDSM community, so take advantage of the resources around you. Learn proper techniques, ask fellow practitioners, attend classes and demonstrations by BDSM educators, and practice skills under the guidance of someone experienced. Learn the risks, the common mistakes that people make, and what is most likely to go wrong. The chance to get some hands-on practice with an experienced person is even better. Don't get tipsy or do drugs, then decide to try out your new flogger. It's just like lots of things in life: Cut yourself some slack. Give each other the benefit of the doubt. Use common sense.

Some players believe in what's called *consensual nonconsent*, an oxymoron and impossibility by legal definitions, but a concept that makes perfect sense to those who subscribe to it. The idea behind consensual nonconsent is that partners don't want to go through a list and map out each and every thing that will happen or consent to activities individually. Rather, they want to state their limits, turn their will over to a Dominant, top, or sadist, and trust in where a scene goes. They want to waive their right to revoke their consent or stop in the middle of a scene. In fact, they agree in advance that something might happen that they don't want or enjoy, or they may be forced to do something that is beyond their comfort zone, and *they're okay with that*. You can read more about this idea in Chapters 15, 16, 18, and 19.

I have seen people push the limits of themselves and their partners. Like the leatherman who used only rope to suspend his slave from a tree. The mistress who used a razor-sharp scalpel to create a decorative cutting on her boy's flesh. Or the daddy who put her entire hand inside a girl's ass. It might sound like scary stuff when you read it on the page, but no one was harmed during those scenes or hundreds of others I've watched. Do you know what is the most common injury at a BDSM conference? A sprained ankle. From *walking*. It's true!

Communication

I'll admit my bias right up front: I think a lot of kinky people are better at communicating their erotic wants, needs, and

BRAIN SEX

I'm walking out of a store, it's late at night. I unlock the car and slide in, shut the door, and suddenly there is a knife at my throat. I can see a bit of the rearview mirror and a figure in black. A rough deep voice tells me to shut up and drive. We pull up at a warehouse and a couple other guys all dressed in black, faces covered, come out and drag me from the car. I fight but it does no good. Someone puts a chloroform rag over my nose and mouth to stop me from screaming and fighting. The world goes dark...

I come to, and my wrists and ankles are bound and something is in my mouth. I can't see anything but I feel cold wires of some kind underneath me. I feel hands all over me, I realize I am in only my bra and panties. So many hands—grabbing, feeling, slapping—and voices insulting me. I feel the sharpness of a knife blade. One of them pulls something off my head, a hood. As I try to focus, still groggy, I see figures. I'm in some kind of dark creepy warehouse. My vision is clearer and I realize I am bound to an old rusty metal bed. The wires I feel are the bare springs of a mattress. I try to scream and can't. As I tug on the binds, I realize it's duct tape and I am not getting out of it.

—KYLIE

Role play and psychological play: animal role play, age play, taboo play, mindfuck, interrogation, objectification, humiliation, kidnapping, orgasm control/denial, forced cross-dressing, medical play

Tools: imagination, costumes, props

limits than a lot of nonkinky people. Notice I didn't say *all*. Communication is a crucial component to an empowered and fulfilling sex life, and it happens to be a big part of kink. People who get lots of play are the ones who are able to say what they want, put it out there, and negotiate scenes and relationships; it helps that within the community there are people around you modeling the behavior and there are workshops on how to do it more effectively. People talk, for minutes, hours, days, or even months, before they play. They negotiate, ask questions, and reveal themselves.

During a scene, communication can be more of a challenge. Certainly you could do a scene where you speak freely and give your partner feedback, like this:

- *Can you slow down a little?*
- *Oh, the cane stings more on my thighs than my butt.*
- *How does this flogger feel compared to the one I just used on you?*
- *I really like the needles in my chest.*
- *That dildo's too big. Do you have the blue one?*
- *You reacted a lot more when the wax came close to your neck.*
- *Shall I adjust the nipple clamps? Can you take them just a little tighter?*

But there may be circumstances that prevent this kind of open dialogue. If you're striving to maintain a strong D/s dynamic in the scene, then a submissive's feedback needs to be more cleverly solicited and spoken. In fact, you can reinforce the power dynamic while communicating. Have the submissive ask for each slap of your hand, count each stroke of the cane, or even beg for the next drop of hot wax. Instruct the submissive to add some "Pleases" and "Thank yous" after each one or make him count each paddle strike. Not only does this move the scene along nicely, it gives the submissive the opportunity to communicate his state of mind. If he begins to wince or hesitate as he speaks, he may be nearing his limit.

Similarly, if you're in a role-playing scene, you want to stay in role. A student doesn't say to the teacher, "Do it harder!" just as a victim doesn't tell his attacker "Please slow down." Plus, (human) ponies and (adult) babies can't talk at all! Or maybe a bottom wants to be taken on a journey, and neither of you want there to be a lot of back-and-forth chat. You want to lose yourself in the rhythm of the flogging, the sensation of the singletail against your skin, or the feet you plan to worship before you. In some kinds of scenes, a bottom is flying so high that he slips into deep "subspace" (a trancelike state some bottoms can achieve, especially in a heavy scene, that often leaves them incoherent). In these situations, eye contact and nonverbal communication are critical. As a top, your ability to read your bottom's body language is essential. Pay attention to the bottom's breathing rate, facial expressions, how his body reacts to sensation, and whether the reac-

INTO THE FLESH

"I don't want any pink ones—that's way too big for me," I told her.

She replied, "Okay, no pink ones." She told me to take my shirt off as she snapped on a pair of blue nitrile gloves.

She rubbed down my chest with alcohol, looked me in the eye with alarming concentration, and told me to take a deep breath. The first needle felt good—a brief prick, then a smooth sliding underneath my skin as the needle penetrated me. I looked down and there it was, a sharp and shiny point that disappeared into a strip of raised skin then came out the other side capped with a blue plastic tip. It was on my chest above my left breast, and it soon had a twin on the right side. She continued moving down my chest, inserting needle after needle. There were some that were so smooth they slid right in with a sensation very much like a finger in a wet pussy. There were some that were slower or deeper and made me squeeze Daddy's hand really hard as she whispered in my ear, "That's a good girl. Breathe. Deep breaths. There you go."

Body modification: play piercing/temporary piercing, suture play, stapling, saline inflation, permanent piercing, cutting, branding

Tools: piercing needles, sutures, sterile staples, scalpels, branding tools

tion changes. Use your judgment about whether something should continue, ratchet up, or wind down.

Aftercare

What happens after a scene is just as significant as what goes on during it. Think about it: you've just had an intimate experience with someone, and you need to make sure she is all right physically and mentally. Whether you play like you have in the past, do something for the first time, explore a new dynamic, or push harder than ever before, it's wise to check in with each other. A scene is like an extraordinary date, a high-flying adventure, or a one-of-a-kind experience—one or both of you are likely to be flooded with endorphins afterward. You might feel energized and excited, worn out and beat down, or, seemingly inexplicably, both. You may be lightheaded or feel like you've run a marathon or seen God. You may feel exuberant, meditative, vulnerable, anxious, giddy, confused, scared, transcendent, or dumbfounded at what just happened. These sensations are all completely normal and quite common. Let the feelings, even the scary or overwhelming ones, wash over you. Take a deep breath.

Imagine you've doled out a heavy caning that tested the limits of your partner's body, pain tolerance, stamina, and perseverance. You just gave it, and good—now take care of the person who took it. If you're the top, part of your responsibility is to ensure the well-being of your bottom. First address some basic needs with questions like these: Do you need to use the restroom? Do you want to stand up (or sit down—because your bottom has been kneeling or standing for an hour during a scene)? Do you want to leave the play space and go somewhere more private, quieter, more comfortable? Are you too warm or too cold? Do you need a blanket or change of clothes? Offer water or another beverage to make sure the bottom stays hydrated and a snack to combat low blood sugar, especially if the scene involved heavy physical play. As part of your negotiation process, you should discuss any specific needs you might have after a scene. That way, you can come prepared rather than scrambling to find an energy bar or a sweatshirt for someone who needs it right away.

Some partners want to process their experiences and feelings about the scene right away, so you need to be prepared to do that; people may have a lot of different emotions afterward. Be ready to listen, validate, and comfort. Some people want sex play, making out, or some sweet cuddling as part of aftercare. Others need a few kind words, a hug, and a lollipop, and they're on their way. After an intense scene, people also like to follow up with a check-in a day or two later; often, right after a scene, you're still in the afterglow, but feelings may come up later that you want to discuss. *Bottom drop* is a common experience where, after the high of a scene wears off (which can take hours or days), a bottom suddenly feels sad, depressed, anxious, lonely, or confused. If you experience this drop, the antidote is often just to reach out to partners, friends, and loved ones for support and reassurance.

Since the bottom is the one who receives the cane strikes, the piercing needles, or the interrogation, there is often a lot of emphasis on the bottom's safety, comfort, and well-being. Do not forget that tops (and Dominants and sadists) also need safewords, have limits, and want aftercare. Tops: make sure you take care of yourself, have what you may need handy, and ask for what you want. Post-scene, tops may experience the malaise of *top drop*, and anyone can encounter *event drop*, which frequently happens after you get home from a fun, play-filled BDSM event. Aftercare is different for everyone; don't assume you know what someone wants—ask.

These definitions are not meant to be exhaustive and definitive; they are a brief introduction to (or refresher course on) common terminology and tenets used in the book. Many of the concepts are explored in depth in the chapters ahead. While it's true that language and labels can often limit, exclude, or box us in, words can also help us define ourselves, communicate, and connect with others. Use these explanations as a kind of shorthand and starting point. It's worth asking others, What does *dominant* mean to you? Why do you identify as a masochist? What kind of a bottom are you? Likewise, ask a play partner what his or her own values are. What do you think about SSC? How do you garner consent? What is your communication style during a scene? Questions like these can lead to useful, fruitful discussions. With a new partner, it's common to get a reference from someone else who's played with him or her. Most kinky people I've met take pride in their skills, experience, and integrity. They strongly believe in the tenets of BDSM, and they are invested in earning the respect of their play partners and peers. Use these conversations as an opportunity to gauge if you are on the same page before you're ready to invest time and trust with someone. If you start with a solid foundation, the sky's the limit.

Endnotes

1. Among those who identify with dominance and submission, many use capitalization in their writing to reflect their power dynamic (as in Dominant/submissive, D/s, Master/slave, etc.). Further, they may capitalize names and pronouns that refer to a Dominant while those that refer to a submissive are written lowercase. For example, a submissive might write: *Mistress is very particular; i hope She appreciates the way i set the table.* In this book you will see both styles, depending on the individual author's preference. I will use the term *D/s* (capitalizing *Dominant* and lowercasing *submissive*) but otherwise adhere to traditional capitalization rules. My goal is uniformity; I do not mean to disregard or disrespect anyone's preferences.

2. Leather Archives & Museum, "Leather History Timeline," http://www.leatherarchives.org/resources/resource.htm, accessed June 6, 2011; Guy Baldwin, *Ties That Bind: The SM/Leather/Fetish Erotic Style: Issues, Commentaries and Advice*, 2nd ed. (Los Angeles: Daedalus Publishing Company, 1993).

3. These lists are not exhaustive; they are examples of some of the activities about which you can find books and classes or that you may see at a play party.

4. David Stein, "Safe Sane Consensual: The Evolution of a Shibboleth," *VASM Scene: The Newsletter of Vancouver Activists in S/M* (September/October 2002); online at http://www.leatherleadership.org/library/safesanestein.htm and http://www.rosecoloredasses.com/SirReal/ssc.pdf. The phrase "safe, sane, and consensual" first appeared in an August 1983 report by members of a Gay Male S/M Activists (GMSMA) committee that was formed to draft a statement of purpose for the organization; it is credited to David Stein, a member of that committee. Stein writes about its origin and unexpected adoption as a community motto in his essay.

5. The term *RACK* is attributed to Gary Switch, who first proposed it on the Eulenspiegel Society's Listserv "TES-Friends" in 1999. Gary Switch, "Origin of RACK: RACK vs. SSC," *Prometheus* 31 (May 1999); online at http://thirstforbdsmknowledge.blogspot.com/2006/09/origin-of-rack-rack-vs.html.

6. Stein, 6.

CHAPTER 2

MAKING AN IMPACT: SPANKING, CANING, AND FLOGGING

LOLITA WOLF

I scanned the play party. Other than a scene going on in the sling, it was mostly clusters of groups socializing on the couches. I spotted the redhead, who was dressed like a doll, with a nametag that said "Dolly." Nobody was playing with her and she did not seem to belong to anybody.

I went over and touched her. She felt so lifelike. I think she was one of those Real Dolls. She was life-sized, but still smaller than me so it was only a little awkward to maneuver her around.

I took her over to one of the less crowded corners. I bent the dolly over my knee. She was a bit stiff, like maybe she wasn't really supposed to bend that way. She flopped over face-first onto the couch.

The dolly wore a short little skirt. First I smoothed it out for modesty's sake and touched her through her clothes. But after a while, I got curious to see what was underneath. I lifted her skirt and she had these beautiful pale-blue panties with a little keyhole detail at the top. Very soft. I fondled her ass through her panties. The dolly was anatomically perfect. Her ass was full and round. My palm wrapped around each cheek perfectly. She was like a custom doll fitted just for me. I became bolder and moved her panties out of the way. I rubbed her butt with my hand. She was so soft, like human flesh.

I sat back and lightly spanked the dolly on my lap and watched the party for a little while. There was a bit more activity and the sling had a group around it. I spanked the dolly a little more intensely and got a rhythm going. I was very happy spanking the dolly. All of a sudden the dolly shuddered a bit. Uh-oh! Was there some kind of internal mechanism that I had jolted? Did I break the dolly?

I don't think anybody noticed anything wrong. The dolly seemed to be working okay again. I decided to pretend as if nothing bad happened. I pulled on the dolly's long red hair until she sat up again. She looked okay and it even seemed that her smile was bigger. Maybe that was just my imagination. I held her in my lap for a while.

SPANKING

Back in the days before I discovered kink, my favorite vanilla sex was rough doggie style. For me, it was more about getting slammed from behind than it was about fucking. That rhythmic pounding felt very good to me. When I finally found the BDSM/kink community, I discovered spanking and my sex life took off.

Some people call spanking a gateway to BDSM, and it's true, many of us start on our kink path with spanking and explore further from there. Other people focus strictly on spanking, and there are whole spanking communities for them, even some who believe that spanking is totally nonsexual. Ack! As for me, I think spanking is the perfect foreplay.

Spanking is great for novices because you don't need any fancy equipment. Some people new to kink can be frightened or intimidated by heavy-duty black leather implements like paddles and truncheons. With spanking, you can just use your hands. It's so convenient.

Some of us get spanked just because it feels good—it's purely about the sensation of a cadenced beating. A good spanking can give you and your partner much pleasure. The goal is not to hurt the receptive partner, but rather to give them an erotic and sensual experience.

Spanking has always had a strong association with punishment: tanning someone's hide is supposed to teach them a lesson, keep them in line, and make them behave better in the future. This can lead to marvelous role play scenarios. You can be a parent, babysitter, teacher, or nun and give your naughty boy or girl a spanking for doing something bad. Or perhaps a spanking is a reward for good service, a ritual to start a scene, or a birthday surprise for your favorite "kid." Public spankings, at a play party or leather event, can be part of a rite of passage—perhaps an initiation to a group or fraternity. Get into the fantasy of it and have fun.

Always communicate with your partner and negotiate a spanking before it happens. Remember, some people are triggered by spanking, punishment, or certain kinds of role play. They may have had bad experiences growing up and spanking may push them to an emotionally dangerous place. Don't force it.

Preparation and Positions

Before you start, set up a good environment for your spanking. The room temperature should be comfortable. Unless you want to set up a role play scenario out in the woodshed, nobody can enjoy themselves if they are shivering. Adjust the lighting. Music can alter the whole scene: for example, a boppy song like Madonna's "Hanky Spanky" will set an entirely different mood than a Gregorian chant. Of course, one atmosphere is not better than another. Add your own touches. Make it your own.

You don't need any accessories or physical preparation for this activity, but it is a good idea to find a position that works for both of you. Get comfortable, because for a nice long sensual spanking you may want to stay in this position for a while. Try sitting on the couch with your partner across your lap. I love what I call the "Princess" position, where I pile all the pillows behind me on the bed and relax propped up like royalty with my partner lying across me right under my hand.

There are other good positions, depending on what you want to emphasize. If you want your partner in a position where you can get access to his genitals, have him bend over a sturdy table or a chair. Or, if you are in a dungeon, there are pieces of equipment like a horse or spanking bench that work well. Maybe your spanking is part of a role play scenario where you sit in a chair and your partner lies over your lap for a traditional over-the-knee (OTK) spanking. If you want to be really strict and give your bottom a physical challenge, have her stand and bend over holding her ankles or knees.

There are also psychological considerations to positioning. You can control somebody by using bondage or holding them down. How you hold them can instill a sense of safety or fear. You can have them present themselves in a manner that reinforces submission or humiliation. For example, responding to your order to kneel on the bed with her head down and her ass up in the air can be very submissive; taking his pants down and letting them pool around his ankles could be humiliating to some people.

And some positions are just more ergonomic for the spanker. What feels best to you? If you need to hit hard, try a position to give you the ability to swing your arm with the most power. And there's no reason to just stay in one position the whole time. It is okay to move around.

Spanking: The Warm-up
A spanking scene should not be rushed. Feel the intimacy. Enjoy this different kind of closeness. It can be especially sensuous if you are both naked. Feel the weight of your partner's body, his skin texture, the way he breathes, the way he moves. Set the tone through intentional touch. For example,

holding someone close to you with your nonspanking hand can give a feeling of being protected and taken care of. Grabbing ahold of your bottom's hair can make her feel dominated or even terrorized.

A spanking can be pleasurable, painful, or both—it can "hurt so good." What can be very confusing is that different people like different levels of sensation. What one person experiences as a medium spanking can feel like a severe spanking to someone else. So, how do we regulate ourselves so that the experience is good? Start slowly!

Warm-up is very important. It prepares your partner. You are seducing your partner both physically and mentally. Rub your partner's butt lightly. Take a lot of time and let him become accustomed to your touch. Move to light pats and escalate very slowly to slaps. If you take your time, your partner will adjust to the heavier sensations gradually. It is very important to build slowly so that your partner will interpret the spanking as pleasure and not as pain.

Communication is very important here. The person getting spanked should be giving feedback. Do you like the sensation? Then say so! Not all audible feedback is through words. Moan. Purr. Giggle. And feedback can be nonverbal as well. Writhe. Wiggle. Raise your butt to meet the spanks. But sometimes the feedback is not so easy to interpret. What if the person getting spanked growls or starts stomping her feet? What does that mean? It could be a reaction that means the spanking is good or it could mean it's too much. The spanker should pause and ask, "What does it mean when you growl like that?" Sometimes the person getting spanked cries. For some people that is a good thing; it is a cathartic way of letting go, clearing the mind, or cleansing emotions. For one person, it can feel really good to cry and keep going; for another, crying means the scene is over.

Everybody has a spanking sweet spot—an area on their ass that feels especially good to them. For most female-bodied people, it is the lower half of the butt in the center. Spanking that spot vibrates straight through to the clitoris. For most male-bodied people, the sweet spot is a little higher, over the anus, where the vibrations go through to the prostate. Some people like it higher or lower on their ass cheeks and may also like spanking on the fronts, backs, or insides of their thighs. Explore and see what feels best to your partner. Spank around her sweet spot and spank directly on it. You can hit all the meaty parts of your partner's body. Avoid hitting over bones, joints, and areas above soft-tissue organs like kidneys.

Take the Spanking to the Next Level

Your hand is capable of imparting lots of different sensations; using them in different ways can vary your spanks. A cupped hand feels completely different from a flat hand. When you use a cupped hand, you are delivering your hit with a soft pocket of air. A flat hand strikes with a bigger punch. Fingers apart gives a more stinging feeling than fingers together. Striking with just the fingers gives more sting, whereas the whole hand gives more thud. Try different types of spanks and see what reactions you get from your partner.

Accessorize for sensation! Experiment with wearing a glove: a soft lined leather glove can add thud; a thin latex glove can add sting. Does your hand get tired or does your partner want more than you can dish out with your bare hand? Try a paddle. Everybody has different preferences: you can choose a leather, wood, rubber, or plastic paddle. My favorite is a leather paddle covered in fur (or faux fur) on one side. It's two sensations in one toy: one side is thuddy and the other is stingy. You don't need to go to a fetish store or spend a lot of money. See what you already have: a big wooden spoon, a spatula, a slipper, a hairbrush, or a Ping-Pong paddle. Try a rubber flip-flop and see what sensations you can create with it—get creative!

As the scene progresses, vary the stimulation. Pause during the spanking to caress your bottom's butt cheeks very softly or use your fingernails to lightly scratch them. You can also add a toy: drag some sensuous bunny fur, a tickly feather, an ice cube, or a pointy letter opener across her butt. You'll be surprised at how sensitive the butt is after having been spanked—every feeling is now magnified. You might get a fun reaction: he may yelp or shudder or squirm.

I love adding a butt plug to a spanking scene. Lightly tap the inserted plug and the vibrations will go all the way through his body. This works best with plugs made of silicone. Spank around the plug, but be careful about spanking directly on it. Depending on the size and shape, it might not feel good. Other people like adding a dildo to a spanking. Again, different people like different things.

Be sensitive to your partner. Watch her body to see how she reacts to different techniques. As you increase the sensation and the scene continues, her breathing is likely to change.

She may wiggle or stiffen. She may make more noises. She may even break out in a sweat. Everybody reacts differently. Again, if you are not sure how to interpret your partner's reactions, ask how he is feeling and what he is feeling. Remember that the same reaction from two different people may mean different things, so don't assume.

Get a rhythm going. Once your partner is warmed up, get into a percussive groove. The beat (yes, that's a pun) should be determined by how your partner reacts, not by the soundtrack you've created. Many people, especially female-bodied people, can reach orgasm just from spanking. For others, it is good lovemaking all by itself.

Some people need a little help to come to orgasm from spanking. Sometimes I reach around with my other hand and spank her clit. The type of spank I use depends on what she likes: sometimes a firm slap or a cupped hand is best. Either way, keep a steady rhythm. With some people I use a vibrator. With a guy, grabbing and stroking his cock can work. Or have your bottom help themselves. Order them to masturbate.

When the spanking is over, keep the connection. Bask in the afterglow, both physical and emotional. Lots of cuddles and hugs. Or more sex! Spanking is great foreplay for other activities like fisting and fucking. Or caning.

CANES FOR PAIN AND PLEASURE

My ex-girlfriend, Peggy, was a great cook. She was also a big masochist. We were well suited for each other. Peggy would make me dinner and I would beat her. After a time, we devel-

oped a little game. I would tell her how terrible her cooking was and then I would "punish" her with a cane, her favorite toy. I would always tell her that I would give her another chance to get it right, and this snagged me another invitation to dinner. There were many fine dinners and many punishments. We even hung a cane in the kitchen so it would be right there for me to use.

One weekend, we traveled out of state to Jack's house. Jack was a bachelor who ate a lot of pizza and Chinese takeout. He was very grateful that Peggy cooked us a fabulous home-cooked meal. The three of us sat down to eat. I took one bite and bellowed, "This is slop! Get me a cane!"

Peggy ran to get a cane. Jack looked down at his food and continued eating. He was totally silent, not wanting to get involved in what was going on. When Peggy came back, I gave her six full strokes of the cane—no warm-up.

We sat back down and continued eating. Jack squirmed in his seat and said in a small voice, "That was role play, wasn't it?"

Peggy and I laughed and assured him that it truly was role play. Jack breathed a sigh of relief and said, "This is really good food."

Now that you are all warmed up and you have your endorphins flowing from a spanking, you may want to try canes. Caning was traditional for severe punishment in the Victorian era and in the British school system, so canes can be the center of some great role play opportunities. Because of their perceived severity, canes have developed a reputation as the "scariest" of all BDSM impact toys, but a caning can be light and sensuous or heavy and painful—it's all about how you wield the cane. Learn how to use a cane properly, build your skills, and you can control the sensations you create. As with spanking, some people get very turned on by being caned and others can orgasm from a caning.

The first order of business is to select a cane. Traditional canes are made of rattan, not bamboo or wood, and should be able to bend significantly. Don't be put off by a cane that is not straight. But while they usually have a curve, canes should always flow in a straight line without any bends. A cane should not wobble when you swing it. You should buy a cane from a store (rather than online or through the mail), so you can test different types. Canes vary in length anywhere from 20 to 36 inches long. Shorter ones are best for novices because they are easier to control; longer ones allow you to hit with more force. The diameters also range from very thin and whippy to much thicker and thumpy. Thinner canes feel stingy and thicker canes feel thuddy. Everybody has different preferences. Some people like both. Maybe they like starting with the thuddy and then moving into stingy after they are warmed up. Check out the tip of the cane to be sure it is well rounded. I also appreciate a comfortable handle. To test a cane, swish it through the air (not too hard or it will break). Does it travel in a smooth line? Give it a quarter turn in your hands and try again. Keep trying until you find the most effective way to hold it. Be sure not to grip the cane too tightly.

Canes are either varnished or left natural. Which one you pick is a matter of taste, but both do require some maintenance. Canes are organic roots from the earth and they dry out. Natural canes need to be treated with water—just soak them in the bathtub. Varnished canes have their moisture sealed in, but sometimes that seal cracks. Just sand the tip and stand the cane up in some linseed oil for a few days, and it will soak up the moisture. You can reseal it with some varnish or clear nail polish.

Canes made from synthetic materials are technically rods, not canes, but they are striking implements, so I include them in the discussion. Synthetic rods are dense, for harder and more penetrating hits. They need a lot less maintenance than canes and are easy to clean. Look for a rod made of Delrin, Lexan, or fiberglass—acrylic rods are more likely to break.

Caning Techniques

Before you hit someone you love with a cane, you may want to practice with an inanimate object, like a pillow. The nap on a velvet pillow can show where your strokes are landing, which is useful for you to see. Or you can use baby powder on the tip of the cane to see where it lands on a dark-colored pillow. Practicing with a pillow can help you to develop your technique and build your confidence.

As with spanking, the traditional position for having your ass caned is bent over. This offers up a nice big target to strike. Caning someone who is standing upright is much more difficult, as there is less surface area. The person receiving the caning could also lie flat on the bed—this can be very relaxing for a serious caning. As in spanking, you want to build up gradually, not too hard and not too fast. If you just start out hitting hard, your partner will likely use her safeword to stop the scene and may be totally turned off to doing any more caning scenes. Warm up with a nice spanking and ease into light taps with the cane. Get those endorphins flowing.

Caning is best on the sweet spot with the lower portion of the cane landing in the middle on both ass cheeks at once. The tip should not go beyond the meat of the ass. The upper thighs—front, back, and insides—can also be caned. The fold between the butt and thighs is safe but can be painful. Stay away from bony areas, especially the tailbone. Do not hit above the top of the ass crack, because there's soft tissue there as well as the sciatic nerve. It is best to hit too low rather than too high, but never so low as to hit the backs of the knees.

When starting a caning session, begin with light taps. Do not use a death grip on the cane. Hold it lightly, so it almost swivels in the hand. As you ramp up the scene, use more wrist action. After a while, you can start using your forearm. Once a bottom is warmed up—and how long that can take is different for everybody—you may be able to do full strokes. Because canes are so flexible, a hard stroke can bend the cane 90 degrees or more. The tip travels very quickly—only a singletail travels faster. Accuracy is crucial: a mis-hit is very painful and can be dangerous. The most common error is wrapping, where the tip of the cane goes beyond the meat of the ass, wraps around the butt, and strikes the side of the hip. Some people don't have a lot of padding there, but regardless, it is not an erotic spot to hit. Wrapping happens because the top's body dynamics change when going from a warm-up to a full strike. The tendency is to move your body, the cane, or both farther forward toward the bottom, which can make the cane wrap. Avoid wrapping by compensating and stepping back a little. Beginning caners can also use padding as extra protection for the person being caned. Put your bottom in a long corset or a weight belt or between two pillows; these accessories and the pillows on either side can protect from mis-hits and wrapping.

When the strike lands, the bottom does not experience the sensation immediately. It takes a while for the sensation to dissipate. The strike lands, there is a little pause, and then the bottom feels it: a hot pain that radiates outward. Timing is key: space out the strokes, or else your partner will go numb and won't feel anything. Wait about 12–18 seconds, before the pain goes away, and then strike again. I like to ask my partners to tell me when the sensation has gone away. You may be surprised at how long it lasts. You can also watch your partner and wait for him to relax his butt muscles. Again, feedback is so important. Watch her move. Listen to her breathing. Deep, careful breathing is good; short, choppy breathing is not. Strike on the bottom's exhale. I like to match their breathing and get into a rhythm.

My favorite way to ascertain how hard the strikes are is to ask partners to rate a hit from 1 to 10. As the scene moves forward, a strike that was rated as a 7 eventually becomes a 3! Vary the strikes. Hit a few medium strikes and then do a heavier one. A snappy blow that is pulled back a bit just before impact will sting more. Follow through past the impact for more thud and penetration. Touch, rub, or caress the butt or genitals between strokes.

As with spanking, you can add dildos, butt plugs, and vibrators for pleasure. One of my play partners likes to rub himself up against pillows while I am caning him in bed. We get into a rhythm: stroke of the cane, a slight pause, and then he writhes against the pillow slowly. Then he gets back into a position where I can cane him again. It's very sexy.

Like rhythmic spanking, rhythmic caning can produce orgasms. Once, during a good caning scene with my girlfriend, I saw her breathing change and her body stiffen, so I backed down. The next day, she told me that if I had kept going, she would have come. I had mistaken her reactions for distress. The next time we played, I watched her and realized that, yes, she was working her way up to an orgasm. I kept up the rhythm and she came.

Sensuous spanking does not usually incur a lot of bruising, especially after a nice slow warm-up, but it can happen. However, most people do bruise from a good caning. Everyone's body responds differently. Some people love the bruises. They are "souvenirs" or reminders of a good time. Some people like to look at them in the mirror or show them off. To lessen bruising, apply cold during the first 48 hours afterward; after that, apply heat. Keep the skin moisturized with some nice lotion. Arnica from the health food store also heals bruising.

FLOGGING

In any dungeon, the most ubiquitous item in BDSM toy bags is the flogger. This toy is popular because it can provide a wide variety of sensations. Most people have several floggers because it's so hard to pick just one.

Choosing a Flogger

Look at the handle. Many traditional floggers have braided leather handles with knots. Does this work look tight and even? Other floggers may have wooden handles. How does it feel in your hand? Does the weight of the handle versus the tails feel balanced in your hand? The length and diameter of the handle should feel proportionate to the tails. Try swinging the flogger to see if it is ergonomic for your body. Decide what feels best to you. If you have small hands, a larger-diameter handle may not feel secure in your hands. Just as a tennis racket should fit your hand and your body, so should a flogger. But not all floggers will fit your body the same way either; picture how a badminton racket feels right yet is different from a tennis racket that also feels right.

Your other consideration is the tails of the flogger. How long should your flogger be? The longer tails travel a greater arc from you. They provide more impact, but also require more strength from you. Shorter tails are often better for beginners because you can have better control for accuracy. A shorter length is also better for tight spaces, like a bedroom with a ceiling fan. If you do acquire a flogger that is too long for you, do not cut the tails: you will ruin the balance of the whip. It is best to trade the flogger with a friend or give it away as a gift.

What material should the flogger's tails be made from? Of course, leather is classic, but there are many kinds of leather.

Deerskin, elk, and lambskin are lightest and softest; oil-tanned leather and bullhide are heavier. Cowhide can range in weight from light to heavy depending on the thickness of the leather. Buffalo and bison are thick but not as dense and give the most thud.

There are also other materials available. Rubber is quite severe. The rubber grips the skin and pulls it away from the body. Bunny fur is light and fluffy. Horsehair is very scratchy (and it's even more intense when wet). Vegans prefer floggers made from plastic or rope. Different people prefer different sensations. Most people prefer "sting" or "thud."

Most floggers have about 18 to 26 tails, but they can range from as few as four up to 150 for a specialty "mop," which is extremely thuddy. The tips of the tails can be rounded or cut diagonally to a point. Pointy tips offer more sting.

Cats have braided tails. They are lighter in weight and do not take as much power to use, but they give a real bang for the buck. The tighter they are braided, the more sting they impart. For greater severity, the ends can be knotted. Flat braids allow more contact with the edges of the tails and can be especially mean.

All these types of floggers feel different. Most people have a variety of floggers so that they can vary the sensation during a scene. They may begin with a deerskin flogger for warm-up, progress to cowhide, and escalate to something heavier. Ask your partner what she likes. An experienced bottom can tell you exactly what she prefers and may even own her own floggers. A novice may not know what he likes, and it is best to start with something light like a deerskin flogger. A deerskin flogger is also very good for a novice top, because you can't do too much damage with it.

The Three Tenets of Flogging

Janette Heartwood was one of the best flogger-making artisans in the country. She taught that a good flogging scene incorporated Accuracy, Intensity, and Connection.

Accuracy

Accuracy means that the flogger lands where you intend it to strike. Practice your swing without hitting your partner. Get a nice smooth consistent "throw." Move an inch closer to your partner and keep throwing the flogger. Watch and estimate where it will land. Adjust your throw so that it will land in the right area. Continue to inch closer until the flogger strikes. At this point, you should be hitting with just the tips. As you move closer, you will connect with more of the "meat" of the tails.

Accuracy is important, not just because you want to control where you hit, but also because it allows your partner to relax and trust you. In order to enjoy the sensation, your partner needs to be confident that you know what you are doing. However, nobody is perfect. You will miss your mark at times. It is important to acknowledge these times. I might say, "Oh, that was a little high. I'm sorry," and caress the area before continuing. This is critical, because if the bottom thinks you did not realize you made a mistake, she'll worry that you will err again. You don't want her to worry about your technique; you want her to relax and enjoy.

Even a very experienced player sometimes hits wrong. I used to really beat myself up about that. And then I played with a very experienced bottom who complimented me on my skill. I remarked that I had hit him high a couple of times. He told me that I had hit him hundreds of times and those two misses made me 99 percent accurate. I have since stopped criticizing myself for not being perfect.

Intensity

Strike gently at first using a short, soft flogger. You can gradually hit harder as you gain skill and confidence. Starting slow also gives the bottom a warm-up, a chance to acclimate to the blows. What feels painful in the beginning may be very pleasurable after the warm-up. Gradually ramp up using longer and either more thuddy or more stingy floggers. Ask your partner if he likes the sting or the thud. Experienced bottoms know what they like; novices will need to try different sensations to learn what they like. Vary your strikes: fast and slow, tips and meat of the tails. Experiment with different ways to throw the flogger. What feels good to you? And what feels good to your partner?

Your partner should be giving you feedback, telling you what feels good and what does not. Remember that much of this feedback will be nonverbal, in the form of body language. Often you can read this body language, but sometimes your partner may move in a way that you can't interpret. It is okay to ask! A movement one bottom makes to process a sensation that feels good, like stamping his feet, could be the reaction of another bottom when it does not feel good. Everybody reacts differently.

Guy Baldwin speaks of a cycle that begins with the top striking. The bottom takes the strike and processes it. Then the bottom responds. Finally, the top reads the response and decides how and when to strike next. This cycle happens very quickly and those who may be watching are unable to see the communication that is occurring.

Connection

Flogging is like riding a bicycle. When you first get on a bike, you are worried about just staying upright. You are overwhelmed with steering, braking, and just getting it to go forward without crashing. After some practice, you begin to really ride—you hop on and stop thinking about how to maneuver the bike. You enjoy the wind in your hair and you're able to take in the scenery. Likewise, once you get comfortable with the mechanics of flogging, you are free to enjoy a flogging scene in which the flogger is simply a tool that enables you and your partner to take an ecstatic ride together.

A powerful flogging is a way to explore strength. It can build confidence and self-esteem through the challenge of taking it, which can be very exciting and satisfying. It can be a means of catharsis, letting go and clearing the mind and the heart. The afterglow of a good flogging is both physical and emotional. Both the bottom and the top feed off this energy that they create together.

Impact play, whether spanking, caning, flogging, or any combination of these, can enhance your sex or just be fulfilling by itself. Try these activities and see how they work for you. It is different for everybody. And it can vary each time you do it.

Author's Note: I learned all this from various people in the BDSM community, and I am still learning. I wish to acknowledge Jo Arnone, Guy Baldwin, Hilton Flax, Janette Heartwood, Conrad Hodson, Michael from Paddles, Constance Slater, and Sharrin Spector.

CHAPTER 3

HOW TO TRAIN YOUR SEX SLAVE

LAURA ANTONIOU

One of the greatest misconceptions in the world of sadomasochism and dominance and submission is the role of a sex slave or pleasure slave. Whenever I meet someone who says they're a sex slave, I know they mean two things: 1) they don't do housework, and 2) they have sex with their top.

Obviously, there's a problem with this definition of sex slave, and that's the absence of the whole "slave" part. Frankly, it's rarely the fault of the would-be slave; they have been clear about their limits and preferences. I am not that fond of housework myself, and if all a top wants is sex, that is generally an easy thing to provide. But let's face it—most adult sexual relationships involve people having *sex* with each other. A sex slave differs from the slave who polishes the silver in that the single most important task of a sex slave is to aid their top in the pursuit of orgasms. Making it kinky, different, and within the realm of dominance and submission is the trick. That's where you—the responsible, clever, demanding, knowledgeable, sexy, and above all, *dominant* top—need to take on the awesome powers of your role. (And, coincidentally, get the best sex of your life, while pleasing your partner or partners at the same time. What a bargain, right?)

First, let's get some concepts organized here. I assume that there is a working adult relationship between two or more people who consent to at least one of them taking the controlling and dominant role: the top (also called mistress, master, lord, lady, dominant, daddy, mommy, Ruler of the Universe, etc.). At least one other person has agreed to take the position of the submissive partner, who has given leadership and authority to the top, and a certain amount of trust. That is the role I call the bottom (also known as the slave, submissive, boy, girl, pet, etc.). People who meander from one side to the other are called awesomely sexy—or, sometimes, switches.

NEGOTIATING WHAT, WHEN, WHERE, WHY

Consent is a primary requirement, one of those big "duh!" items. But you also need to negotiate what your arrangement will look like. Is this a full-time thing? Does it only apply to weekends when you are together? Is it limited to a certain list of behaviors and themes and to certain times and places? How much time can the top reasonably require the bottom to give to this training, considering other responsibilities and restrictions on their time? Can the top punish the bottom for missing the mark, and if so, how? The more parameters you talk about before you start, the fewer times you will need to put up the "time out" signal and have a "What the fuck was that about?" conversation. No one wants to have those.

In your negotiation, you should both understand why you want to start a sex slave training program. The first—and best—reason should be to have better sex. Other good reasons might include the romance of dominance and submission, the excitement of playing with power, the fun of role playing, the satisfaction of learning something new and discovering these things together. In a world that is unfair and often arbitrary and cruel, the ability to escape into the timelessness of our erotic relationships is priceless; a system where excellence and goodness are rewarded and correction and punishment are given with trust and affection is an added bonus. So, talk about it and come up with some reasons why you want to train a sex slave, why your slave wants to be so trained.

You probably think you know what sex is. Here's the working definition I use: *Sex is any activity that increases the potential for orgasm.*

Pick up your jaw. Surely you didn't think sex was limited to "When two perverts love each other very much, the boy pervert puts his penis into the girl pervert..."? Once you expand sex beyond heterosexual procreation, it can get deliciously tricky. Yes, blow jobs are sex! So is cunnilingus, anal sex, fucking between the thighs and between the tits, and hand jobs. So is telling your partner a story while she uses a vibrator. So is a long spanking, Japanese bondage, dancing the tango, masturbation, dirty talk—you get the picture.

We can't limit ourselves to activities in which orgasm is always or even usually achieved. If we relied on that definition, many women never have sex while being vaginally penetrated. Also, those with limited sensation in the lower genitals might never achieve orgasm, and yet feel pleasurable sensations from sexual activities.

Already, the potential for being a sex slave is growing—can you see it? A sex slave should aid in any activity that increases the potential for the top to have an orgasm. But it's still not a complete picture, because it is missing the single element required to make it work—the *active* and *controlling* role of the top.

"But all I want is for them to have sex with me when I want to!" This is the usual cry from tops who are not quite sure what to do with someone as wonderful as a potential sex slave. This is not entirely about a lack of imagination: for many people, a partner or two who will have sex with us any time we want is enough of a fantasy to make for many happy years. The challenge—and part of the pleasure—for a good top is not only to enforce their sexual will upon their loving slave *when* they want sex, but *how* they want it. This is made possible by a training regimen that includes exercises, assignments, rewards, and punishments.

Training is by its very nature an act of authority and dominance. Tops should strive to use any tool they can to evidence their authority; otherwise their slaves will wind up running things. Don't believe me? Sit back and wait, and you will see how many slaves cheerfully take control of a situation. If that makes you happy, and it makes them happy, you can skip this chapter and move on to another topic. But if you want a more structured relationship where the top is actually applying dominance and the bottom is actually submitting to the top's authority, give training a try.

Dominant/submissive relationships and play styles are a very common kink, and subject to a lot of misinformation. Do not be misled by well-meaning people who tell you that you need to be full-time, 24/7, total-power-exchange, whatever the new trend is, to do it "right." The tips in this chapter are guidelines—use them the way you might use a recipe on the back of a box of spaghetti. It might work for you as is—or you might want a dash more basil, fewer pine nuts, or a ton of extra cheese. You need to make the relationship that fits you and your partners best, not the one that sounds good in Internet chat rooms. Whether you do this to spice up date nights, on alternate weekends, only when on vacation, or anytime you can find the energy and privacy, just make sure you do it when it makes you happiest.

EXERCISES AND ASSIGNMENTS

The first step in training a sex slave is to identify your ultimate goal. Yes, "The slave should please the mistress at all times," sounds very nice in the abstract, but strive for specific goals on a more narrow track. Training, like the rest of our kinky relationship styles, is above all *personal*. Never try to use someone else's training program! What do they know about your preferences, your style, your relationship, your lovers? Nada, zilch, zip. Using their training would be like using their underwear; it might look like it fits, but wouldn't you rather have your own?

So, start out with something you enjoy, a pleasure your slave might become better at providing. Let's say a mistress really enjoys having her pussy licked, and her slave is adequate at pussy licking, but perhaps not inspired. The goal is to get the slave up to speed on cunnilingus.

Next, the top determines what *exercises* you can use to improve the slave's linguistic talents. Of course, some exercises will be personal and sexual: "Lick me there. Harder. Swirl your tongue. Now, suck my clit." These instructions, delivered while the slave services the top, are the most obvious start of a training program. You can also deliver instructions before you practice the act. "Using your tongue like a brush, spell out all the words to 'Bohemian Rhapsody' on my clit, and suck on my labia during the instrumental parts."

But there's no need to stop there. How about including others in the training? If you are polyamorous or nonmonogamous, bring in a special teacher, or someone to practice with, or on. Or bring in some inanimate teachers—dildos to stand in for cocks, little candies for clits, pillows and balloons for skills in beating, shaving, body painting, whatever floats your boat. Due to the restrictions on nudity and sexual behavior in public, sexuality educators have found many ingenious ways to demonstrate erotic techniques on and with objects. Feel free to use their tricks for your own training program. Of course, you can also send your slave to attend classes and workshops given by others and report back to you on what they learn. An order to learn something is an *assignment*.

Assignments can be brief and amusing, like "Find ten slang terms for cunnilingus." They can include more serious research, as in "Read this book on anal sex and fisting." Or they can consist of directions to practice a technique: "Massage five people at next weekend's fetish frolic." They can be geared toward a specific act, or even to a style of behavior. Suppose you and your partners love the fantasy of an Edwardian household, complete with high teas and fancy clothing and strict master/servant roles. Assign your sex slave to find the right clothing, and set the scene for the grand, formal tea-service-and-caning you schedule for your next big date night. Or have them read some nice Victorian porn to you, posed on their knees while you sip your tea or brandy.

When training expands beyond the realm of sexual techniques and encompasses role playing and other behaviors, the world likewise grows tenfold. Suppose it's not just the sex and play and fucking the top enjoys, but the attitude of the bottom that makes her so much more ecstatic. Maybe you enjoy a cringing, fearful victim for your diabolic schemes as opposed to a fancy-free happy slut! Or, perhaps the formality of the whole "Yes, my lord and master" role play is more to your taste than "Sure, honey, right after I worm the cat." Either way, giving the bottom an order to behave the way you like for a set amount of time is a great way not only to use that authority of yours but to set yourselves up for some great flirting.

Flirting? Why not? Flirting should not end just because

you have an established relationship. And erotic role play, whether full-time or fit-into-your-busy-lives-whenever-you-have-the-time-and-privacy-to-enjoy-it, is flirtatious, sexy, and its own reward. So tell your slave, "On Saturday, all day, I will be holding you captive; tremble and obey!" That is an assignment that should be received with pleasure and anticipation. The worst that can happen is a few giggles. These can be survived.

An important thing to remember when developing training exercises around role playing and fantasy games is to make sure everyone is on the same page. Parent/child role playing is very popular, whether it's a naughty boy getting spanked over Mommy's knee or Daddy's precocious little slut trying to find out what happens when she does *this*. But if the Daddy in question wants a precious girly partner who will climb on his lap and kiss him shyly and tease him with her white panties, but the little girl in question wants Daddy to sneak into her bedroom at night and hold her down in the dark while saying terrible things—this will not be a good date, let alone an example of good training.

REWARD AND PUNISHMENT

The next step in developing your personal training program is to figure out what to do when your slave 1) does things wrong, and 2) does things right. *Both* of these are fun and will improve your sex and play and enhance your dominant/submissive roles.

Your two responses are called *punishments* and *rewards*, and yes, I meant it when I said both are fun. If you are not having fun doing something in your relationship, then don't do it! One thing some people seem not to understand about these ways of enhancing our lives and our partnerships is that they are all optional; none of them should be a burden. And this includes the scary concept of punishment.

Remember, the goal of your training program is to improve your sex life and enhance dominance and submission. Your submissive partner already wants to please you, and already gets pleasure out of doing so, as a volunteer. The ability to punish him for doing something wrong is what shows that you, the top, are the one in authority. It also shows that the top is *paying attention*, which is perhaps even more important. Everyone likes to be the center of attention—bottoms more than most people, even if they insist otherwise.

Suppose the bottom has been engaged in a strict training program in toe sucking, also known as *shrimping*. This specific fetishy behavior can be very tricky to master, despite seeming sort of obvious. (Take toe into mouth. Suck. Repeat.) Problems can arise, however, if the toe suckee is also ticklish, or likes specific tonguing behavior, or wants special attention paid to one toe over the others, or wants a massage with the hands at the same time, or, well, anything else. One fine and sexy night, the bottom forgets the vital instruction to cup the top's heels in both hands while lovingly laving the little piggies. When the top comes out of her postorgasm stupor (if she gets that far without this critical bit of stimulation) she can announce with glee—or dire and stern mien, if that's her style—that the bottom, having failed to be completely pleasing, is now subject to punishment.

This point in the scene is a good reminder of why partners need to complete their consent and negotiation way ahead of time. But even if the bottom draws the line and says, "Nope, no hitting me or making me stand in the corner. No one puts Baby in the corner," for whatever good reasons he may have, the top can usually come up with some way to express a negative and dominant reaction to an error or failure that does not bring up bad memories, make the bottom feel dumb or unattractive, or in any other way betray the positive and sexy aspects of their relationship. For some people, it's as easy as "Do it again, slave!" Or it might require more creativity, such as: "To make amends for your toe sucking catastrophe, you will have to attend the next chick flick/action adventure movie with me and not whisper a single catty thing during the whole show." Believe me, they'd probably prefer that you spanked them.

If, however, spanking (or other sex and play activity) is on the table, punishment becomes what I call "another excuse to play." If your relationship is more formal, make the punishments very different from what you use for fun. Bring out the canes if you normally use your open hand, or the steel handcuffs if you normally use the soft leather cuffs. Make it quick and complete, and include a chance for the bottom to beg for mercy (because that's hot), then offer forgiveness, smooch or otherwise soothe, and move on to greater efforts at improvement. For many people who enjoy the submissive role, being punished is one of the times when they feel authentically submissive—they are accepting something they'd rather not have. This expression of their obedience is paradoxically very rewarding. Many bottoms report that after being punished, the moments of discomfort and embarrassment actually turn to memories they embrace with pride and affection, or even reenact in whack-off fantasies. Just make sure that all your play is not punishment—that will just lead to deliberate disobedience to get sexed up. Not that there's too much wrong with that—*if that's what you intend.* But if you want a more positive training experience, you have to use the next item on the list of training tools: a reward.

The other side of the punishment coin is *rewarding* your bottom. Rewards can be anything the bottom likes, ranging from "Do it again, slave!" to accompanying them to the next chick flick/action adventure movie and not making too many catty comments during the show. Or, for that matter, a spanking. You can even get tricky and reward him with a new assignment. But whatever reward you use, make sure it's accompanied by some verbal praise and affection and you will find the light of pleasure and adoration shining all around you. For obvious reasons, rewards are less tricky to negotiate than punishments—you will rarely run into a reward that might stir bad memories of toxic parenting or dismal school days. But it's always a good idea to know exactly what the bottom likes, lest you announce a reward that he might accept with a raised eyebrow or giggles. Beware of "Homer Simpson" rewards: Don't give your slave a bowling ball that fits your hand—get him a butt plug that fits his ass.

BEING CREATIVE

Eventually, even the most jaded of tops might find that they seem to have trained their bottoms in everything they want. This is usually a combination of laziness and lack of imagination. Why should you stop refining pleasure? Expand your training to more variations. When your sex slave has become the world's most amazing cocksucker, start him on ass licking. Or, even better, assign *him* to find some new variation on cocksucking that is not currently in his repertoire. But be specific, so as not to look completely lazy. "Go learn something to please me" has got to be the worst cop-out tops use after "Go on the Internet to find the slave protocol." Either way, you get what you deserve. Remember, this is all personal, and direction and leadership comes from the top. Give your slave what she needs to get her started! And if by chance you are very vague, accept what she offers with an open mind and good grace, and resolve to be more specific and dominant for the next assignment.

Keep in mind my definition of sexual behavior. It's not just what gets you off, it's what gets you in the neighborhood. Does a long, slow dance make you horny? Then having your slave become a good dancer is a worthy goal. Does having your back scrubbed with scented salt crystals in a hot shower make you more ready to turn around and fuck someone against the tiles? Then having the scrubs available—and the slave ready to hop into the shower with them—is part of what you might want to train them to do. And you can get more esoteric too—perhaps the slave should shop for new scrubs, or merely keep your favorites in stock. Or even *make* you some, if they are crafty that way.

While not limiting yourself to genitalia-based service, don't box yourself off from the pleasures of receiving other SM-like pleasures. Many tops honestly enjoy a long, sensual beating or even a short and painful one. They just confuse the act of receiving pleasure in that way with being submissive. There is a huge difference between submitting to a lashing and ordering someone to beat you harder; knowing this and being able to enjoy whatever you like is part of what it means to be a confident, strong top.

Sadly, many dominant people have also deprived themselves of the pleasure of being fucked or sucking off their slaves because of the misconception that these things make them appear submissive. It is not the act which is dominant or submissive, but the attitudes and intentions of the partners that makes it so. "So, slave, have you earned the right to fuck me?" can be the most empowering, dominant thing a top can say, reducing the lucky bottom to a quivering mass of erotic flesh. Or it can merely be one of the slave's many sexual uses; it's *your* slave, after all. Their hands and cocks are yours, just as their mouths and other holes are. What use you make of their bodies and their skills is part of their sexual service to you. And if your new slave is unlearned in the art of top-fucking, lucky you: here is a brand-new opportunity for more training, more assignments, more rewards and punishments.

TESTING

One aspect of training you might also use for fun and profit is *testing*. I don't include it as one of the basic concepts because, really, every time you have sex can be construed as a sort of test. But you can plan specific tests, whether you announce and schedule them or spring them on your slave with gleeful surprise. You can use a test to mark the end of a training period, or just to spice up a quiet weekend.

Say your sex slave has been blacking boots for three months now because having your boots done makes you so crazy sexed up you need your slave to learn every detail in order to make your boots sparkle and your wobbly bits eager. You can either announce the quiet evening at home with that treasured pair of boots you've withheld from him these long months, or you can set up something at your local leather bar with all your friends and family on hand to watch and celebrate. Your slave does the boots, you grab him and fuck him on the floor in the basement, or right there on the pool table in front of that gang of friends. He passed the test, yay! It's happy all around.

Or, you've been having your slave learn the most advanced and esoteric fisting techniques for quite some time and you think she's ready to give you the ride of your life. But instead of setting up the home dungeon with the sling and the candles and the soft music playing, you are waiting for her with heels in the air on the dining room table when she gets home from work. "Do me, slave," you command. "Make it good, or it's back to fingering cantaloupes for you."

Training a sex slave does not lead to your normal pop quiz, that's for sure.

Finally, remember that your training relationship is ultimately only a small part of your human interaction with your partner; it's not required, not vital, and certainly not something worth making each other unhappy about. If it causes you to fight, or hurt each other's feelings, suspend it and take care of what really matters first. Keep in mind that your goals are to expand your sexual playground, increase your erotic connection, enhance your intimacy, and embrace the complex and exciting aspects of dominance and submission. If these are foremost in your intentions and you can laugh at an occasional mistake without feeling threatened or diminished, your role as the leader and teacher, judge and arbiter, administrator of rewards and punishments will be all the more satisfying, both to you and your sex slave. And your slave will thank you for it. Exactly the way you prefer!

CHAPTER 4

WHOLE HAND SEX: VAGINAL FISTING AND BDSM

SARAH SLOANE

When I slip my hand into my partner's cunt, my entire focus narrows down to the feel of her vaginal walls around my hand: tight, hot, pulsing, and slick. I don't feel the rest of my body—I only feel the point of connection between the two of us.

—CHERYL

I never really thought about fisting until I was in my late 20s and just beginning to fully explore my sexuality. I came across some fisting porn on the Internet and really couldn't see the point in it; it looked scary, painful, and decidedly unsexy. It took me a few years to get past my preconceptions about it; one day, it just clicked for me. Now it's one of my favorite activities with new partners and long-term lovers alike, and every time I get the chance to be inside one of them it's an entirely new experience for both of us.

As a fister, I get a feeling of exultation from penetrating my partner with a part of my body that is attached to me (something that I don't otherwise have the ability to do). I love the feeling of my partner's heartbeat through her vaginal walls; I love feeling the slickness of her body, the tightness around my hand, and hearing her expressions of arousal and exertion. I love helping her work toward the goal of my hand inside her; it feels like midwifing a spiritual experience, watching and exhorting her to take just a little more, breathe just a little deeper, relax and let the orgasm come. Fisting is a singularly spiritual and carnal experience, and it's one that brings amazing intimacy with it.

Fisting is not a BDSM-only activity; yet, the combination of power, control, energy, and sex that it offers makes it a natural way to explore power exchange. It can affirm a bond between partners, requiring and building trust between people in a way that few other types of play can do. And it can be incorporated into almost any type of scene, from humiliation to reward to bondage to beatings, and even into spiritual guidance and growth.

Fisting is often misunderstood, not only because of the images that often spring to mind when talking about it (the old idea of "punch fucking," for one), but also because we are generally not used to exploring the internal organs with as much mindfulness as is necessary to create a sexy, healthy scene. So, let's start by taking a look at the physiology of the vagina.

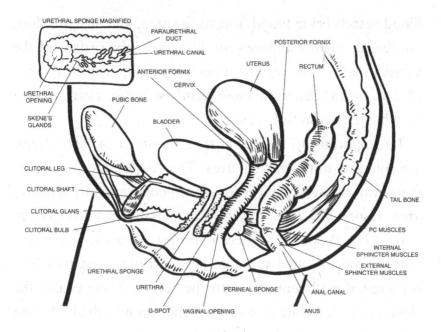

Illustration 4.1. Female Anatomy

PHYSIOLOGY

The vagina is a muscular tube that connects the cervix with the exterior of the body. (See Illustration 4.1: Female anatomy. It may be helpful for you to refer to this as you read through the next section.) It's a multifunctional organ—it does everything from encouraging ejaculation during intercourse to passing a baby from the uterus into the world. The urethra and the glans of the clitoris are located just above the vaginal opening. It's all protected by the labia majora and the labia minora, which cover the vaginal opening. While some people have smaller labia than others, everyone's labia are very sensitive, and they can be one focus of stimulation during fisting. The entire vulva is a highly vascular area; a large number of blood vessels bring blood flow to the area, and a tremendous number of small capillaries are just under the surface of the vaginal tissue. This density of nerve endings, especially in the clitoris, means that even small, gentle sensations can create a very big impact in this region.

It's important to remember that a number of other things are going on in the vaginal area. The G-spot, located on the front wall of the vagina, is for some people a highly sensitive area, responding especially well to pressure from fingers or hands. The A-spot (or anterior fornix) is another especially sensitive area, located at the deepest part of the vagina where the vaginal wall connects with the cervix. There is also the structure of the clitoris, which reaches up into the body and surrounds the vaginal walls. Visualizing the various anatomical areas when fisting can help you create more specific sensations and even stronger orgasms for your partner.

A word about pronouns: For consistency's sake, I've chosen to use female pronouns to refer to the person being fisted. However, I recognize that people of all genders can have vaginas, and I encourage you to use the pronoun(s) that apply to you.

> *I never had an orgasm from fisting until one of my previous dominants decided to use a Hitachi Magic Wand on my clit while he was pressing upward on my G-spot. The combination of being absolutely filled by his hand, along with this unstoppable vibration on my clit, connected the two sensations in a way that I'd never experienced before—I felt like he was pushing my G-spot up toward my clit, and the orgasm that happened (along with the resulting ejaculation) took us both by surprise. Fortunately, I've been able to make it happen again and again, and it's even added to the ways that I can come when I'm playing on my own!*
>
> *—LAUREN*

Vaginal walls are relatively stretchy—they are designed to allow for childbirth, after all—but there are a few factors that can affect the elasticity of the vagina and therefore a person's ability to be fisted. The three main limiting factors are hormones, surgery, and bone structure.

Estrogen levels are part of what helps the vagina to remain elastic; those with a low level of estrogen, whether as a result of menopause, hormone therapy, or other causes, will find that the longer their estrogen level is low, the thinner and less elastic the vaginal walls become, and the more likely they are to tear. They may additionally find that they have problems with dryness and irritation due to a lower level of vaginal lubrication, which may make penetration more painful. There are a number of treatments for this, including estrogen suppositories and creams, that some people can use to reduce the irritation and help the vaginal walls retain more of their elasticity. Regardless of what treatment is used, when you know that your partner has lower estrogen levels, make sure to use plenty of lube, and choose lube that is less likely to contain irritants. And take plenty of time to warm her up.

Those who have had surgery on or around the vagina may also experience challenges with being fisted, primarily due to the presence of scar tissue. Scar tissue does not stretch like the skin that it covers; additionally, the skin around it may be weaker than usual. To help avoid pain, take care not to place too much pressure against the scar tissue—again, use plenty of lube. A number of women have had their vaginas created or altered through surgical means; while they may not have the natural stretchability of other vaginas, it is possible to fist them. The key to this is how much these women dilate and how much they engage in penetrative play; those who do either or both regularly are more likely to be able to receive a lover's hand. However, this is one of those cases where your mileage may vary; even those who do stretch regularly still may not be able to get a whole hand inside them.

There is also build and bone structure to consider. Some people are "built small"—they may not have the ability to take a fist without a lot of work, if ever. Some people find that being fisted is very easy. In general, women who have given birth have an easier time with being fisted, as the ligaments in their pelvis loosen somewhat and are able to accommodate larger objects.

Together, all of these factors—as well as psychological and physical comfort—contribute to how easily someone can be penetrated with larger objects, including fists; by being aware of these factors and working with them, we can plan our scenes to be more pleasurable and longer lasting.

I've never been "successful" at being fisted. Even people with very small hands haven't been able to get in all the way—but the feeling of fullness of even just four fingers is so erotic to me, and puts me in such a submissive head space, that "getting it all the way in" just isn't that important to me anymore.

—KATHLEEN

COMMUNICATION AND EXPECTATIONS

Fisting is one form of BDSM and sexual play that requires active and ongoing consent on the part of the recipient. It is very difficult to fist an unwilling partner; it's also possible to do damage to someone's vagina if she doesn't communicate pain or discomfort to you. Furthermore, a successful fisting scene is a cooperative effort; the top and bottom need to be in communication about what is working and what isn't, including things like whether there is enough lube, or there is a pinching sensation, or even whether the bottom needs to change positions. Finding a way to encourage this communication even in situations where there is a formal power exchange agreement is integral to the success of the scene and to the well-being of all participants.

A word about "success." Many people feel that their fisting scene is not successful unless one partner has penetrated the other up to the wrist; if they haven't, then it's not a successful scene. Wrong, wrong, wrong. Just as everyone's body is different, everyone's body has different capabilities on different days. It's not at all unusual for a regular fisting bottom to have a day when it's just not working; likewise, sometimes even the most challenging vagina will open up to an object much larger than usual with little to no prep work. Often, our bodies show our stresses. If a bottom is worried that she will not be "good enough" if she can't take her partner's entire hand, she may not be able to relax enough to let it happen. Fisting is about the journey, not the destination. I've had scenes where I could only use three fingers on my partner that were far more physically and psychologically satisfying than scenes where my whole hand disappeared in under 10 minutes.

PREPARATION

When you're getting started with your fisting scene, there are a few things you'll want to have on hand. A high-quality lube is of primary importance; I recommend lubes that are glycerine and paraben free, as they are less likely to irritate vaginal tissue, but any lube that feels comfortable for the bottom will work. Some people prefer silicone lubes and others prefer water based; either of these is fine for vaginal use. I would steer clear of oil-based lubes, which can trigger yeast infections or other irritations. During fisting, the vaginal walls are more stressed than in most other kinds of penetration, so it's very important to select the best-quality lube you can find to protect the tissue from abrasion and irritation.

I also highly recommend gloves, even for partners who are fluid-bonded. Our hands have a number of small rough spots, including hangnails, calluses, and dry skin, that can scratch and scrape the vaginal tissue; with a gloved hand you create a safe, smooth surface for fisting—it's like the world's most perfect sex toy! Both latex and nonlatex gloves are available; I prefer to use nitrile gloves (a nonlatex material), as they are unlikely to cause irritation to my partner and tend to be stronger than latex gloves. If you have longer fingernails, I recommend either clipping and filing them or tucking small bits of cotton ball into the fingertips of the gloves to cover your nails and keep them from feeling sharp for your partner.

If possible, I also recommend placing an absorbent underpad or towel underneath the fistee. A really good fisting can be messy; with lube, ejaculate, and other bodily fluids, it's easier to plan for a mess and not worry about it later. A vibrator is another handy tool to have; many people like to have their clitoris or anus stimulated during a fisting scene.

> *I've gotten to the point where I've made the preparations for a fisting part of the foreplay. I text her from work to tell her to get the supplies out, and she knows how I want everything laid out. I have her get out the wrist restraints (we like her hands to be held back to keep her from being able to touch herself) and turn the temperature up in the bedroom so it's nice and warm. By the time I get to her house, I'm worked up, she's already turned on, and the scene has started before we even touch.*
>
> —PAUL

Relaxation is the key to fisting. Having the bottom in a position that relieves the tension on her legs and hips goes a long way toward helping her open up to your hand. For some people, this may mean that they are most comfortable on their back with their ankles propped up in ankle straps on a sling or on their partners shoulders (my personal favorite); for others, it may mean that they're lying on their side, or on their belly, or even on all fours. Trying a few different positions, even changing it up in the middle of the scene, can offer a lot of insight into what works—especially when it gives you an opportunity to slip your hand in at different angles and adjust to the changing physiology of your partner.

Some people like to use chemical means to help relax: "poppers," a glass of wine, some pot, or another substance that they feel helps them ease into being fisted. Unfortunately, when we take chemicals to relax, we also lose some of our ability to feel and respond accurately to sensations that may be the precursor to injuries. Part of being risk aware is both understanding and acknowledging the risks of playing in a particular way; we take steps to minimize or eliminate as much of those risks as possible. With fisting, it's worth giving some thought to and discussing whether it's a good idea to be under the influence of any mood-altering substances, legal or illegal, that may have wide-ranging repercussions for either partner's health.

TIPS AND TECHNIQUES

When getting started, remember that arousal goes hand in hand with relaxation in the process of getting fisted. Someone who is turned on, who wants to get fisted, and feels excited about it is far more likely to enjoy the process than someone whose body is pushed to go from zero to 60 in three seconds. Just as with any other form of BDSM or sex play, we need some time to get our bodies warmed up. Other kinds of kinky play can do the job—a flogging or caning for someone who enjoys those sensations, or perhaps a bit of bondage and humiliation. Of course, you can also do some more direct sexual stimulation with hands, mouths, toys, or cocks, as well!

As your partner gets more and more turned on, start using your fingers or penetrative toys to get her vagina more relaxed and opened up. My preference is to use my fingers, slipping them in slowly, one at a time, and letting my partner's body get accustomed to the sensation before adding an additional finger. I find that taking lots of time, letting my fingers slowly stretch the vagina out rather than thrusting in and out, most often gives me better results; the thrusting can often fatigue the vaginal walls and be overwhelming for the fistee, especially over the course of the play date. I have a number of friends who prefer to get their partners ready to take their hand by using different-sized dildos or vibrators to stretch the vagina, then move on to inserting three or four fingers and working up from there. Again, each body is different, so take time and ask questions to find what works best for you and your partner.

The bottom may mention that she feels an urge to urinate—this is perfectly normal and, in fact, may be the precursor of ejaculation. I know that the first few times I had a partner try to fist me, I worried so much about not peeing on them that I remained too tense to really enjoy the session. Having absorbent pads handy to catch any urine that comes out can help; mostly, it's vital for you to reassure your partner that she can relax about it, or even encourage her to "push" with the feeling of needing to pee, since that often triggers ejaculation. Above all, it's vital not to overreact or immediately pull your hand out and shuffle your partner off to the bathroom; the feedback loop that we create with a partner when we express upset or disgust about their bodily functions will eventually limit their ability to relax and enjoy the scenes we create with them.

> *I like to feel dirty when we play, so sometimes my Mistress tells me how wet I am, or how I look with my legs up in the air and my cunt open for her. She'll encourage me to squirt, tell me to bear down, not just because it makes it easier for me to orgasm, but also because She knows that it's both embarrassing and erotic for me. For some reason, when She calls attention to what my body is doing, it makes it easier for me to just go with it and enjoy it.*
>
> *—JEN*

Stimulating the G-spot or A-spot can help the bottom relax and enjoy the sensations even more; in some cases, orgasms that happen during fisting can create more relaxation postorgasm, allowing you to fit even more of your hand into your partner. However, for some people the additional stimulation actually pushes them to a place where they tighten their vagina even more, so pay attention to whether different kinds of stimulation get your partner more into the fisting or take her away from the experience that you want to create. If you want to increase the G-spot stimulation, pressing or rocking your hand to push against it with your thumb or forefinger can work well, as it doesn't require you to remove your hand in order to add to stimulation. Some people also enjoy tucking a small bullet vibe into their hand and pressing it against the G-spot.

As you gradually insert more of your hand into your partner's body, check in regularly. Ask your partner to tell you how it's feeling, and where she's feeling pain or discomfort. This is really important, because it will allow you to adjust your technique to help her feel more comfortable. You may also have her use hand signals like the universal "stop" sign (holding up her outstretched hand) or a thumbs-up if she's ready for more—this can provide an additional way for her to communicate while still being able to stay in the moment. Also, remember that it's important to relube your hand regularly, and check your gloves for any signs of breakage.

Many people get frustrated during fisting. "I can't get my hand in past the knuckles" or "I'm out of room" are frequent comments from novice and sometimes even experienced fisters. The reality is that we are working to fit our hands into a part of the body that usually doesn't expand more than a few inches in diameter, so it's not always the easiest thing to make happen. The first "bump in the road" is often just before the knuckles enter the vagina—we run out of "stretch" and may feel as if we are totally blocked.

There are a few ways you can work past this. First, make sure your partner is relaxed and is doing what she can to open up to you. (More about that in a few paragraphs.) Second, slowly rotate your hand, gently pressing in at different angles and in different positions as you go "around the clock" in your movements—often there is a particular angle or direction where you'll feel a bit more room to work with. It's not necessarily intuitive—one of my partners can't take my hand if it's parallel or perpendicular to her, but she can easily let it in if my hand is at a 45-degree angle. You may also want to try those different body positions I mentioned earlier. Some people find that being on their hands and knees (doggie style) or lying on their side relaxes their pelvic muscles and allows them to take even more. The good news is that once you've found a great position, chances are it will continue to work for you in the future.

When the challenge isn't so much the stretch to accommodate your knuckles but the length you have to work with, it's time to adjust your hand position. Fisting doesn't happen effectively unless we use our hands as flexible tools, and visualizing your partner's internal landscape through your touch can help you adjust your position to get more of your hand inside her. I like to close my eyes and "feel" for opportunities to curl my fingers; in most cases, the vagina opens up past the first few inches, and you can begin to curl your fingers to make a fist. Usually the thumb, once it's inside your partner, will naturally fold in toward the center of the palm; letting your fingers close around it will help you penetrate more fully and fill your partner's vagina more completely.

FOR THE BOTTOM

For a bottom, the experience of fisting is almost as much a mental as a physical process—perhaps even more. Being able to allow our body to open up to our partner is not an easy thing for many of us, so learning techniques to help it along is key to your own enjoyment—and it makes you an active participant in the process, which is even hotter than just lying back and waiting for it to happen. Start by focusing on your own relaxation—this can be difficult if it's your first time or if you're in an unfamiliar location, but it's absolutely key to being able to accept your partner's hand. One technique I use is deep breathing, which helps our bodies relax more fully with each breath. As you breathe deeply, focus on the muscles in your lower body—your vaginal muscles, your ass, your hips, even your belly—and imagine that each muscle relaxes just a little bit more every time you exhale.

Another way to open up is to use visualization techniques. A simple one? Continue to breathe deeply as I described above, but shift your focus specifically to your vagina. With each exhale, visualize your body opening up more and more. As many of us already know, our minds have an amazing influence over our bodies (including functions that we don't often consider to be linked to our emotions), so use your creative juices along with your sexual juices to have a more incredible experience being fisted.

The one thing that will almost always defeat us in our search for pleasure is a negative attitude. Expecting that you will be able to easily take your partner's entire hand, or that you will orgasm from the experience, or even that you will be able to maintain your composure, can short-circuit your ability to go with the flow of the experience and appreciate it for the process that it is. While you're breathing deeply, stay focused in the moment. If you feel happy and full of laughter, let it out; if the sensation brings up sadness, or fear, talk it out (or cry it out) with your top. Our bodies have their own memories; it's not uncommon for sex and kink (especially when they push our previously conceived limitations) to tap into some of those memories. By releasing them, we can embrace our own internal reality and give our tops the opportunity to create that safe space for us as we experience them—and move on toward even more pleasure!

Discomfort is part of the process for many people when they're being fisted. Let's face it—a part of the body is being stretched pretty wide open. Pressure is a common feeling; breathing and relaxation techniques should help you process and move beyond it. However, you should alert your partner to a sharp pain or burning sensation as soon as possible. The vaginal walls are quite strong in most people, but they can still be damaged with small tears to the tissue—and that means you will have both pain and healing time, as well as, potentially, scar tissue that can make future penetration less comfortable. This is really not an area where putting up with pain for any length of time is a good idea. Often, you can manage it by letting your partner know where the pain is, as much as you're able to, and having her adjust the angle or amount of pressure behind her penetration to a more comfortable level.

The end goal of a fisting—whether it's with the whole hand in up to the wrist and multiple ejaculations, or just getting to the knuckles for the first time—is to heighten the sense of intimacy between partners. When a top has his hand inside his partner, not only does the act say, "I own this," but it also provides the rush that comes with reaching a new plateau with his partner; the sense of control, power, and physical intimacy can be overwhelming. The first time I really experienced this was after a few hours of off-and-on insertion play, finally ending up with my knuckles just getting inside my lover's body. She started orgasming, and I could feel her vagina hot and tight, squeezing my fingers together—but rather than feeling uncomfortable, it felt like I was an active part of her orgasm, not just the person who was doing the work to get her there. I felt mentally and emotionally aroused to an incredible degree—I had a brain orgasm right along with her physical one. Since then, I've looked at fisting a partner as a great honor and privilege, and it's become one of the most pleasurable tools in my arsenal of sexual domination.

AFTERCARE

When is the fisting scene over? When you both say it is. I've had as many fisting scenes end because of my own hand and arm cramps as because my partner was finished. It should go on as long as you both comfortably want to continue. Some people like to finish off with an orgasm (or two, or three, or a hundred); some people like to stay at a plateau for as long as possible and then slowly bring the scene to a close. There is no right way to do a fisting; as long as neither partner feels that the end was abrupt or unpleasant, then you've done it correctly.

You may see some blood as a result of the fisting; this is not terribly uncommon, as the capillaries that run close to the surface of the vaginal walls may break open and leak a small amount of blood. However, if you see larger amounts of blood, you will want to back off and make sure that your partner is not bleeding from damage to the vaginal walls. Minor bleeding will subside very quickly and is nothing to be alarmed about; if it doesn't stop quickly or increases, a trip to the doctor or urgent care is strongly recommended.

As part of aftercare, you can use witch hazel wipes (the kind made for hemorrhoid treatment) externally to soothe any swollen tissue around the vulva; they will also remove the excess lube gently. I also recommend that the bottom urinate as soon as possible afterward, to push out any bacteria that could cause a urinary tract infection. Spend time connecting, emotionally and spiritually, whether it's cuddling, having more sex, or going out to dinner and sharing a dessert. This helps bring a natural close to the intensity of the scene. The aftercare may be a bit different from what we think of as a post-BDSM scene, but the end result should be the same: both (or all) parties involved feel comfortable, connected, and cared for.

Like most BDSM activities, vaginal fisting is a physical activity that can, at its finest, bring about an amazing sense of self, of connection, of esteem and pride, and most important, a feeling of power for everyone involved—not just the top. To open up one's body and offer it to another is the height of strength and trust. To be the person who is invited to enter should be embraced with humility, compassion, and joy. Fisting is transcendent sex. If it is done in a way that honors all participants, it can take us on a journey to the farthest reaches of our growth as sexual, kinky beings.

CHAPTER

5

BONDAGE FOR SEX
MIDORI

Bondage sex is hot. Your senses are heightened and the mundane details of life melt away. You can savor your lover's every touch and movement as forbidden fantasies come to life and pleasures are intensified.

Bondage is one of the easiest and most versatile forms of kinky play. It can be as simple or as elaborate as you wish it to be. Whether your tastes run sweet and romantic or gritty and intense, there's bondage fun to suit your different moods. It's just as much fun in your bedroom, a romantic getaway hotel, a fully equipped dungeon, or even an alpine tent. The creative potential and sensual possibilities are endless, making this the perfect pleasure art for a lifetime of boredom-proof sex. So it's no surprise that bondage is one of the fastest growing trends among the sexually adventurous.

THE PLEASURES OF BONDAGE

What is it about bondage that draws your attention? Do you fantasize about it? Does your lover? If you've tried it before, what about it got you off? If you've not tried it, what sort of fun do you imagine it to be? Knowing what makes you and your sweetie curious about bondage is the first step in creating an amazing experience. This is something I constantly emphasize to the students in all levels of my workshops. It can be easy to get caught up in the technical details, bogged down by the variations or wonders of the equipment, so keep your focus on why it's hot for you.

Each person's answers to the *why* of bondage will be different. When I ask my readers and students why they love to play with bondage, the reasons they give are wide-ranging and diverse. The list below is just a sampling of examples that come from real people. Run through it alone or with a partner. How many are on your list? On your partner's? Do you find yourself thinking of completely different reasons that aren't listed here? Simply going through this list of things that other people love about bondage may be an excellent way for you and your lover to discover new things about each other.

- A lover's surrender into sensual captivity, fulfilling fantasies of romantic helplessness
- The thrill of being naughty and breaking taboo

- Escape from daily responsibility
- Thrill of anticipating the unknown
- Full-body relaxation while receiving erotic attention
- Erotic humiliation
- Sensation of full embrace
- Firm bondage in a quiet atmosphere over a long period can create a sense of inner peace and meditative stillness
- Bondage as part of erotic role-playing games lets you unleash your dirty evil genius, hot sex slave, or any character that turns you on
- The physical catharsis and excitement of being able to thrash about as much as one likes
- A change of pace from one's usual sexual routine or play style
- You can appreciate the beauty of the bound body or allow your own body to be exhibited as you're bound
- The intimate pleasure of giving or taking control with someone you feel a deep connection to
- Immersion in deep trust and emotional intimacy
- Pleasure in the sensations of rope, leather, or other bondage gear on the skin

- Expression of sensual creativity

- Bondage positions and equipment that touch or bind against erogenous zones just perfectly, increasing turn-ons and intensifying orgasms

What other reasons you can think of? Knowing the root of your bondage pleasure will also help you select the right equipment and technique. Why struggle with a truckload of exotic toys if all you need is a blindfold?

BONDAGE BASICS

Regardless of the type of bondage play you want to explore, there are some basic preparations that you have to consider first. Think of it as your preflight checklist.

Up for It?

Talk with your lover and make sure you're both into giving it a try. Even if your sweetie likes surprises, just springing bondage on them mid-sex can be disastrous. Discuss what each of you wants to try; make sure that you're clear about your desires and where your limits are. No need to make it sound like some boring legal arbitration, make it a flirty, dirty hot talk!

If you've never chatted about this—give the conversation time. Your partner might have hesitations and concerns. Hear them out and compassionately address their concerns. Remember that it can be intimidating to try a new and taboo sexual activity. Remind them that this is about fun and pleasure.

Top or Bottom?

Decide who's going to be the one binding (usually called the top), and who's going to be bound (the bottom).

The Escape Clause

Agree on a safeword or safe signal. Having one is especially important if you're playing fantasy role-play sex games. Sometimes it's fun to play at saying "No!" but your partner will feel more confident in the games when they know what the real "NO" sounds like. Tops also get to use a safeword if they don't feel comfortable with what's going on. Once you set a safeword or safe signal, respect it and abide by it. Solid trust is the foundation of fabulous bondage.

Oops Tools

Sometimes things don't go the way you planned and the bondage needs to get undone quickly. Sometimes your plans for smooth unbinding go awry. Sometimes equipment fails. Have your "oops tools," or contingency tools available. Emergency medical shears, which have rounded tips and cut easily through a variety of materials, are an essential part of your bondage toolkit. You may often hear them referred to as EMT (emergency medical technician) shears, and they're available in most drugstores. They are great for rope, leather, cloth, tape, rubber, and other materials.

If you're using devices that lock with a key, have several spares available. When using multiple padlocks, take the precaution of using locks with identical keys. Spare keys are a lot easier to hide and carry than giant bolt cutters, as well as being far more stylish.

Sweet Aftercare

How you wrap up your bondage experience is just as important as how you do the wrapping. Aftercare is what each participant wants and needs to transition from bondage play to everyday life. When you finish a delicious bondage experience, it's like being in an altered state. Great sex in all forms can be like that. Rushing out of it can be jarring at best, and at worst it can put you in an intensely bad mood for a while. That happens often enough that it's called a "drop." Both bottoms and tops need aftercare, so schedule your play time with that in mind. How long it takes and what constitutes aftercare varies from person to person. Here are some examples:

- Sex
- Cuddling
- Talking about the fun you just had
- Being quiet
- Chocolate
- Time together
- Time alone
- Snacks and water
- Putting the tools away
- Ignoring the tools for now

Have the Right Tool for the Job

Gather the toys you want for play. This includes the bondage equipment as well as any sex toys, extension cords for vibrators, lube, pillows for propping up the body, slings and sex swings, and any other items you might want. I'd hate for you to be all tied up with the lube just out of reach! Don't forget to turn off your phones before play, and select your bondage toys according to what feeds your appetites. I've listed below several varieties of toys and types of play for you to consider. You can also skip ahead to the First-Time Scenarios I've created for you.

TOOLS: DIY FUN AROUND THE HOME

No need to spend a fortune! DIY bondage is one of my favorite hobbies. Look around your home, in hardware stores, or even dollar stores and you'll be in bondage heaven. Here are just a few ideas:

Scarves

Long scarves are fantastic as blindfolds, wrist bonds, and ties to bedposts. They even make a great dildo or vibrator harness. They're easy to wash after play. Bathrobe belts and stockings are great, too. If you want to keep it green, recycle your old sheets by cutting them into bondage strips. Here are some scarf ties that we do in my Wrapped for Pleasure class:

Simple Scarf Wrist Tie

Equipment
1 scarf

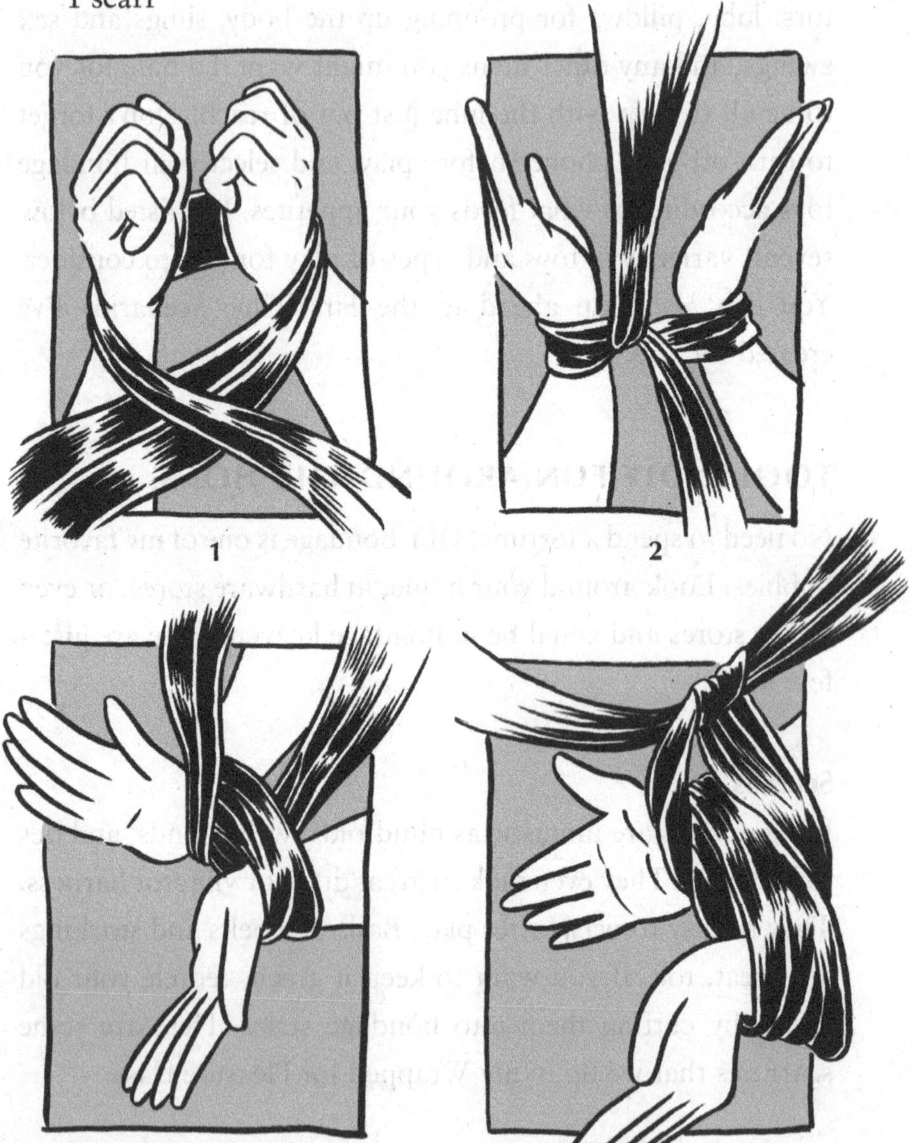

Illustration 5.1. Simple scarf wrist tie

Directions
1. Bring the wrists together, separated by about an inch. Drape the scarf across the wrists. The midpoint should be between the wrists, with both ends hanging down.
2. Bring the two ends together below the wrists, and cross them with a twist, bringing the scarf parallel to the wrists. This is not a knot, just a twist.
3. Bring the two ends up, one between the elbows and the other between the hands.
4. Tie the two ends together in a simple overhand knot, just as you would to start your shoelace tie. If the scarf is slippery, you can tie one more overhand knot.

THE SIMPLE SCARF SCENE

Ingredients
    you and your lover
    2 long scarves
    your favorite sex toys, lube, safer sex supplies, and whatever else you enjoy in your usual sex life

Action
Bring the scarf out long before the sex fun starts. Use it to tease and suggest all the fun both of you will have later.
    The top gently blindfolds the bottom. Make out!
    Tie the wrists together above her head, behind her head, or behind her back. It's up to you and how you like to shag.
    Shag! Slow and sweet or rough and wild, it's up to the two of you.
    Give aftercare lovingly.

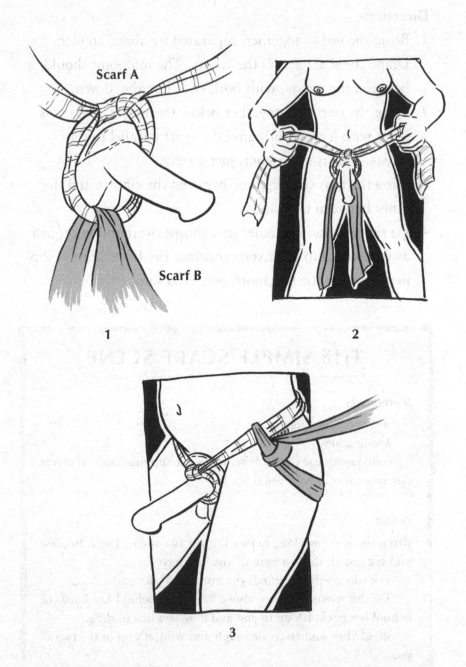

Illustration 5.2. Midori's dildo harness

Midori's Dildo Harness

I invented this harness because I got tired of ill-fitting commercial harnesses. This is a fantastic harness—it's secure, easy to clean, fits anyone, and travels well. Men can use it to sport a second cock above the one that they grew themselves!

Equipment
1 favorite dildo with flanged base; 2 scarves (suggested length: multiply hip measurement x 1.5. Example: 40" hips x 1.5 = 60" scarves)

Directions
1. Take Scarf A and make a loose overhand knot (which I refer to below as "That Knot") at its midpoint.
   Take Scarf B, place through That Knot, bisecting Scarf B. Scarf B will now have two hanging ends of equal length.
   Insert the dildo into That Knot.
   Tighten Scarf A and That Knot firmly around the dildo.
2. Tie Scarf A snug and low around the hips. It's easiest to tie this in front, with the dildo at the back, and then turn the scarf around. Very important that it be snug.
   Place the dildo in the desired position on the body.
3. Take one end of Scarf B, hanging from the dildo, and pass it between the legs and under the butt cheeks, ending near the hip bone. Tie onto Scarf A near the hip bone.
   Repeat with the remaining end of Scarf B.
   Test the harness all over for security.

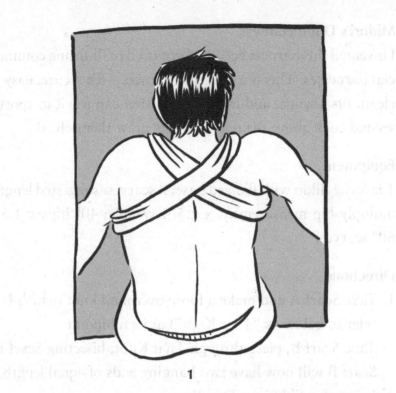

1

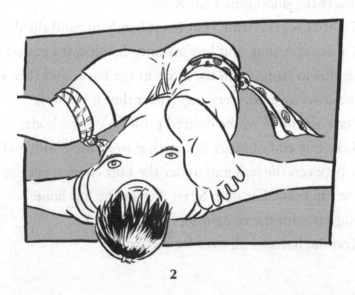

2

Illustration 5.3. Scarf sex sling

Sex Sling

Equipment
2 short scarves and 1 long scarf

Directions
1. Take one short scarf and tie a band around one thigh, just above the knee. This should be snug but not tight enough to hamper circulation.
   Do the same with the second short scarf on the other thigh.
   Tie one end of the long scarf onto the right thigh band. Have the bottom sit on her butt with her legs out and knees up. Have the bottom hug her knees. This is important for a fabulous shagging position and comfort later.
   Lead the free part of the long scarf from the right thigh over the right shoulder and pass under the left arm.
   Pass the long scarf under the left thigh band and pull through fully.
   Lead the remaining length of the long scarf from the left thigh over the left shoulder and pass under the right arm.
   Pass the long scarf end under the right thigh band and tie off with a simple overhand knot.
   The long scarf should make an "X" pattern on her back.
2. Have her let go of her knees. Gently lean her back. Her legs will be held up and apart by the scarves.
   You can easily move her back and forth and up and down by holding the long scarf where it attaches to the thigh bands. Add the wrist tie to this and you have a fun and easy sex bondage setup.

Other Items

- *Sleep masks:* Best stealth blindfold that you can take anywhere.

- *Leather belts:* Strong leather belts with many holes to adjust positions are the best.

- *Cling wrap:* Ordinary plastic wrap used in the kitchen makes for fantastically easy and fast bondage. No knots or buckles needed. Use safety scissors to remove it quickly or to create holes when you want access to your lover's good bits. Slip a vibrator or an ice cube between layers of plastic wrap, just on the right spot, and drive him crazy.

TOOLS: LEATHER AND METAL

Leather

Leather fetters are truly classic bondage toys and they're fodder for many people's fantasies. Leather is supple and friendly on the skin, and the texture or scent alone can send some people into a state of intense arousal. Many sex shops have a kinky section with leather restraints. Quality varies widely. If at all possible, inspect the items personally. I like padded restraints, as they make it easy for a long night of passion. Look for the following qualities:

- Sewn well with strong thread
- Leather edges that are finished smoothly or tucked under the stitching

- Properly dyed so the dye doesn't rub off and doesn't smell funny—strange smells are often signs of an improper or toxic dying process
- No rough edges
- No unfinished or sharp edges on any metal hardware attached to the restraints
- Correct size for the person it's intended for

Tug the fetters and pull on all the parts as if in actual use, especially the connecting hardware. See if all the parts hold together.

Wrist and ankle restraints are the most common, but there's a vast range beyond that, from blindfolds, thigh cuffs, arm restraints, and hoods to full body bags that have access points for the naughty bits. I highly recommend shopping at the Stockroom and Mr. S Leather for quality restraints.

To start with, get wrist and ankle cuffs that separate easily with simple clips. This makes it a cinch to change positions. Use a short length of chain or even a scarf to separate the limbs and attach them to the bed frame for a sexy spread-eagle sex tie!

Metal

Bondage equals handcuffs, right? Wrong! I love playing naughty cop games in the bedroom as much as anyone else, and I do have a few pairs of handcuffs. They're fabulous for the visual effects, but sadly they're not so good for actual bondage, especially if you're just starting out. They're hard on the skin and body, often causing cuts, bruises, and nasty pinches, or worse. Novelty-store handcuffs are worse, as they keep tightening down and have nasty rough edges. A few great uses for metal handcuffs: put them in a box with a card as an invite; wear them as a prop; use them as connectors for leather restraints. And if you're feeling especially perverse, a pair of handcuffs can serve as an interesting cock ring.

Other metal toys specifically designed for bondage are generally much safer. Look for strong welds and a smooth surface. For wrists and ankles, look for wide band-style cuffs. Wrapping the wrists, ankles, and any other tender places with sports wrap before play is another way to ensure comfort in your fantasy cruelty. Look for products from reputable manufacturers. Of course, you can go DIY and use a length of high-quality metal chain with padlocks to create a fierce-looking and very effective restraint.

Other Materials

Bondage lovers are ever inventive, so just about anything can become a potential toy. Any material that turns people on will get turned into restraints. Other materials that can be used for good bondage include wood, spandex, canvas, neoprene, latex, rubber, PVC, ACE bandages, cast plaster, yarn, fur, tape of all sorts, and even specialized medical restraints.

ROPE BONDAGE

Rope is my first love in bondage play! As a college student, I was inspired by the memories of watching heroes and villains being tied up on the TV shows I watched as a child in Japan. Additionally, the economic realities of being a student put expensive gear hopelessly out of my reach. What began as necessity became a passion, leading me to study rope bondage thoroughly and develop my own unique philosophy and style. The books that I've written and the weekend-long Rope Dojo workshops that I teach to this day are a result of that early passion. Nearly three decades later, rope still makes my heart skip a beat.

Rope is endlessly versatile, whether you can barely tie your shoelaces or you've memorized the entire *Ashley Book of Knots*. Don't let yourself be intimidated by thinking that you have to know fancy knots. If you like complicated, that's great, but you don't need to know them.

Selecting the right material is key. Cotton rope is fantastic for beginners. Look for it in magic stores and better sex stores. Avoid the nylon, polypropylene, and most other synthetics, as it's easy to cause rope burns with them. Hemp, jute, raw silk, and bamboo ropes are lovely, but they're quite expensive. When you're starting out, stick to shorter lengths of 12, 15, or 20 feet. Nothing kills a hot scene like the top getting tangled up in his or her own rope.

Here are a couple of simple ties to use on single limbs or a pair of limbs:

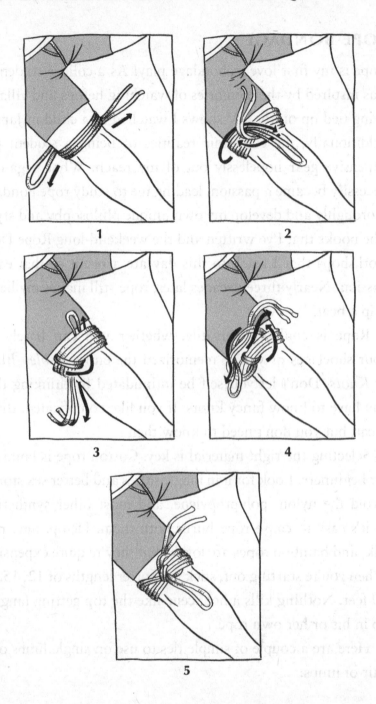

Illustration 5.4. Simple single-column rope tie

Simple Single-Column Rope Tie

What's a column? Think of the body as a series of columns—the wrists, ankles, thighs, and torso are all columns. A single-column tie is very useful. It works just like leather cuffs or belts as a foundation for binding one part of the body to another, or to furniture.

Equipment

1 piece of rope (10' or so for wrists; longer for larger body parts). Cotton ropes are great!

Directions

1. Double the rope.
   Wrap the doubled rope around the column of your choice. About three times is sufficient for most wrists and ankles. If you want more coverage, make more wraps.
   Make sure that the looped end, also known as the bight, is not too far from the wrap. Six to eight inches is a good length.
2. Cross the loop and the loose ends.
3. Tuck the loop end under the wraps and pull through to the other side.
4. Tie an overhand knot with the loop end and the loose ends.
   If the rope is slippery, as many synthetics can be, tie an overhand knot one more time.
5. The loop can be a convenient attachment point for other ropes or hardware such as carabiners or double-snap links.

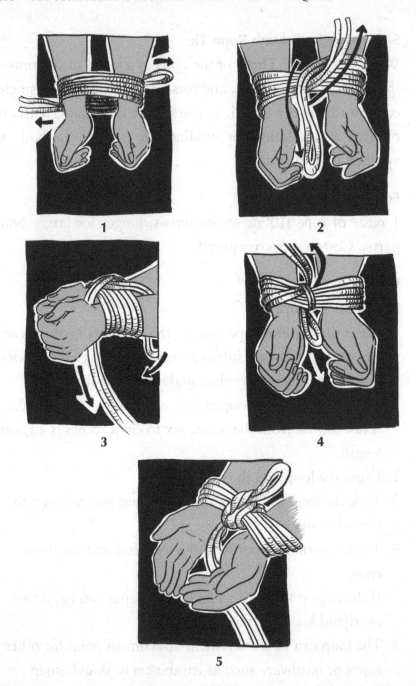

Illustration 5.5. Simple double-column rope tie

Simple Double-Column Rope Tie

Tie two body parts together with one rope!

Equipment

1. The two columns should be held a couple of inches or so apart.
   Double the rope.
   Wrap the doubled rope around the columns of your choice.
   About three times is sufficient for most wrists and ankles.
   If you want more coverage, make more wraps.
2. Cross the loop (the bight) and the loose ends. It's not a knot, just a twist. These two ends should now be perpendicular to the wrist wraps.
3. Drop the two ends on opposite sides of the wrap.
   Wrap both ends a full rotation. They should now be back up on the original side.
4. Tie an overhand knot with the loop end and the loose end.
   If the rope is slippery, as many synthetics can be, tie an overhand knot one more time.
5. The loop can be a convenient attachment point for other ropes or hardware such as carabiners or double-snap links.

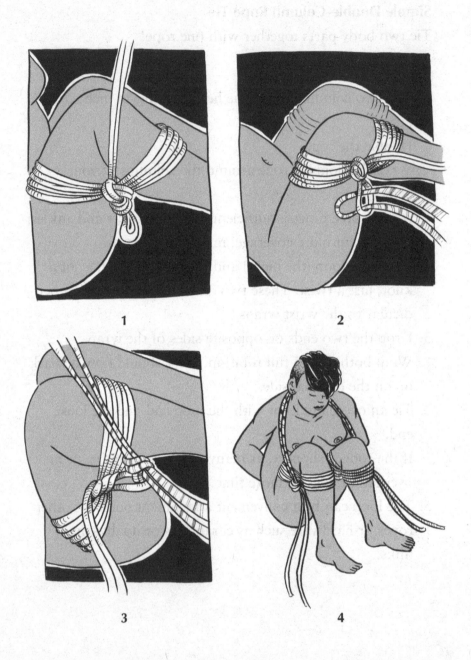

Illustration 5.6. Open-leg crab variation

Open-Leg Crab Variation

Equipment
3 pieces of rope (20' to 25' each should suffice).

Directions
1. Bend one of the bottom's legs so that the ankle is tucked to the thigh. Tie a double-column tie between the base of the thigh and the ankle. Repeat with the other leg.
2. Tie the third rope to the loop end of one of the double-column ties.
3. Wrap the third rope around behind the back and run it through the loop on the other double-column tie.
4. Adjust the spread of the legs to taste. Tie off with a simple overhand knot.

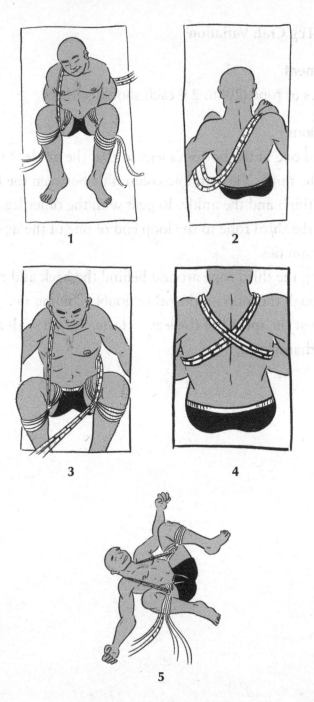

Illustration 5.7. Rope sex sling

Open-Leg Crab Variation Detail / Rope Sex Sling

Equipment
3 pieces of rope (20' to 25' each).

Directions
1. Set up two double-column ties, as in the basic Open-Leg Crab tie.
   Tie the third rope to the loop end of the double-column tie on the right leg.
   Have the bottom hug his knees. This is important for a fabulous shagging position and comfort later.
2. Lead the free part of the third rope from the right leg over the right shoulder and pass under the left arm.
3. Pass the third rope through the left column-tie loop and pull through fully.
4. Lead the remaining length of the third rope from the left leg over the left shoulder and pass under the right arm.
   Pass the third rope end through the right loop and tie off with a simple overhand knot.
   The third rope should make an "X" pattern on his back.
5. Have the bottom let go of his knees. Gently lean him back.
   His legs will be held up and apart by the ropes.

Japanese-Style Rope Bondage For Female or Male Bodies

Here's an interesting body harness, or a *karada*, based on a Japanese-style rope bondage form called *shibari* or *kinbaku*. This harness works well for men or women—just adjust to each person's contours and features. This is a very simple version. For a more fully detailed version, see the harness in my book *The Seductive Art of Japanese Bondage*.

Equipment
1 long piece of rope (50' to 75', depending on the size of the person)

Directions
Find the midpoint of the rope.

Drape the rope around the bottom's neck, with the midpoint at the back of the neck and the ends hanging down the chest.

Tie the two ropes in front of the body in a simple overhand knot. Try to place this at the mid-chest. Make sure it's not too high—you don't want it to press on the throat. This is Front Knot 1.

Tie another knot around mid-torso. You now have Front Knot 2

Tie the third knot at the lower belly. This is Front Knot 3.

Run the two lines between the legs and bring them up to the back.

Tie a knot at the lower back. This is Back Knot 3.

Moving up, tie the next knot at the mid-back. Now you've made Back Knot 2.

Tie the last knot, Back Knot 1, at the upper back.

Run the two lines through the loop at the midpoint of the rope.

Separate the two lines. Run one under each arm to the front of the body.

Run the two lines between Front Knots 1 and 2 and pull through. Separate the originally vertical lines so they form a diamond.

Pass the ropes toward the back on either side of the torso.

Run the lines between Back Knots 1 and 2 and pull through. Separate the originally vertical lines so they form a diamond.

Repeat this process down the body, forming a new diamond shape below each knot.

At the end, tie each end off with a simple overhand knot.

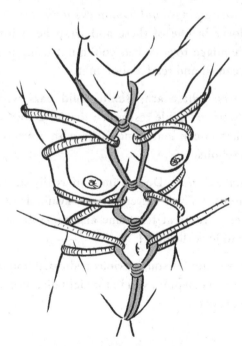

Illustration 5.8. Japanese bondage

FURNITURE AND ACCESSORIES

While there are specialized bondage furniture makers around, most of us don't have a dedicated adult playroom or dungeon, so we make the most of what we have. Walk around your home and see what pieces of furniture would be strong enough and fun to use as a bondage frame. If you're shopping for regular furniture anyway, give it some good pushing and shoving to test for bondage compatibility. Here are a few ideas:

Beds: Not all four-poster beds are sturdy enough for raucous bondage sex. If yours is wobbly, don't use the posts as tie-down points or you may risk pulling them down on you and your sweetie. Some people have their beds custom-made with bondage in mind. If that's not in your budget, you can always get a well-built wooden bed and sink eyebolts into the hidden part of the frame.

Sex slings, love swings, and hammocks with freestanding frames: Put your lover in one of these and wrap her with any of your preferred bondage toys. When you're not using it as a bondage frame you can sit and read a book in it.

Spreader bars: These are usually solid bars with attachment points for wrist or ankle restraints; they're great for keeping the legs spread. You can make one easily with a wooden pole and a couple of eyebolts.

Door bondage devices: Door frames are really strong, so why not put them to use? These clever devices, available at many quality SM suppliers, are great for home and romantic hotel getaways. Remember to lock the door!

When you're ready for some serious dedicated bondage furniture, drop me a line. I can point you in the right direction for your home dungeon makeover!

TYPES OF BONDAGE

Now that you know some materials and toys, let's consider a few of the different styles of play you can use them for.

Sexual

The objective here is a good shagging and righteous orgasms. For sexual bondage, first visualize what position you want the bottom to be in, and then restrain him in that position. Make sure that all the good arousing body parts are accessible. It would be sad if you worked really hard to get him bound and then realized you couldn't get to anything.

TIP: BODY POSITION DURING ORGASM

How does the body arch and tense during orgasm? Do the feet point or curl? If you want the person bound to achieve orgasm easily, bind their body, especially the legs and feet, into the posture they assume during orgasm. If you want them to have an intensely challenging time achieving orgasm, then bind their legs and feet in opposition to their usual mid-orgasm posture. This curious little tidbit is one I discovered through years of dedicated "research."

Fantasy Role Play

Could a pirate's-wench fantasy or cops-and-robbers scene be complete without bondage? No! Pick the right bondage tool to fit the fantasy. Ye olde pirate's wench wouldn't be bound in futuristic medical devices, would she? Don't be surprised when your fantasy role play bondage turns into sexual bondage.

Escapology

Escapology is the challenge and pleasure of escaping from clever, well-executed bondage. If the escape artist bottom is any good, he will get out. Period. If you're the top, their escape doesn't mean that you failed, so don't be discouraged. Your objective is to make it as difficult, challenging, and time-consuming as possible. Bring out the stopwatch, scorecard, and any distraction you can think of!

Predicament

Predicament bondage is another favorite of those tops and bottoms who love challenges and puzzles. In my class on this topic, I define predicament scenes as bondage that limits or controls mobility by intentionally creating conflicting desires. For example, imagine your lover on all fours with clamps on her nipples connected to the headboard in front of her. At the same time, labia clips (or for a man, a cock ring) tied to the footboard board pulls her gently back. She has to find the spot with just the right balance as you sensually tease her all the while. Don't be surprised if there's more than a pinch of masochism involved in it as well.

Sensory Deprivation and Mummification

Some find a deep state of calm and meditative peace in bondage. For these people, it's a deep and quiet altered state where all the mind's chatter about mundane life disappears and they take a minivacation. To make this possible, reduce sensory input. Using earplugs, headphones, and blindfolds, you can eliminate all sight and sound. Noise-cancelling headphones are a particularly effective addition to your sensory depravation fun. Hoods, mummy-style wrapping, and bondage body bags (called sleep sacks) will reduce the skin sensations. At all times, make sure that they can breathe without obstruction.

YUMMY MUMMY

Ingredients
- blindfold
- earplugs
- cling wrap
- emergency medical shears
- old bedsheet or giant beach towel
- ice cubes
- candles—plain paraffin candles are best. You can find these in grocery and general stores in tall glass containers. Don't use fancy candles made of beeswax or containing other ingredients, as they have a higher melting point and can cause nasty burns.
- match or lighter
- bottom's favorite sex toy or vibrator
- bottom's favorite sensual foods

continued on page 118

Action

Blindfold the bottom and insert earplugs in her ears.

Spread the bedsheet or towel on the bed.

Take the cling wrap out of the box. That cutting edge is evil!

Light the candle and place it somewhere safe but reachable.

Stand the bottom with her arms hanging down along the side of her torso, then begin wrapping her body from the shoulders down to her knees. (Tip: Don't start with the feet! If they get unstable it's easy for her to keel over.)

Sit or lay her down on the bed.

Continue wrapping from the knees down to the feet. If you like, wrap the feet.

Lay her in the middle of the sheet or towel.

Slip the ice cubes between the layers of cling wrap alongside the nipples, genitals, and other fun places.

Drip candle wax on the cling wrap in fun places.

Alternate the ice and wax for fun.

Place the vibrator or sex toy where she'd like it. Use the cling wrap to keep it in place.

Surprise her with her favorite sensual foods while the ice, heat, and vibration is driving her wild.

Tear away the wrap to get to the sexy bits.

Enjoy!

Give aftercare decadently.

Self-Bondage

Like so many forms of sex, bondage can be enjoyed alone. But no one is there to fix a mistake or rescue you from a mishap, so risks are increased. The solo bondage player needs to be careful to have a way out. In case of any emergency, make sure you can move one hand easily to free yourself, and have your oops tools nearby.

RISKS AND REALITIES

Bondage has its own risks. As I tell my rope bondage students, "Dead bottom, bad bondage. Bad top, no biscuit!" Always heed the advice of *The Hitchhiker's Guide to the Galaxy*: "Don't panic." With common sense and a little planning, most disasters and bad scenes can be avoided. The bottom is responsible for alerting the top of early signs of any possible problems. Bottoms can be reluctant about this. I know some of you worry that as a bottom you should just let the top do their top thing, but trust me, a good top wants to know. Think of it this way: if you can let your top know of a possible issue, they will make the necessary adjustments and the pleasure can last longer for both of you. Not telling them is not nice and considered poor SM etiquette.

WHAT TO AVOID
Boredom

Boredom is a scene killer. Tops who spend too much time fidgeting with the gear bore many bottoms to death. Bottoms who focus on just their own pleasure bore the motivation right out of most tops.

Rope Burn and Gear Chafing

Hot spots, rope burns, blisters, and chafing really distract from the fun. Prevent rope burns by moisturizing the skin, and exchange your synthetic rope for soft cotton and other natural ropes. For metal, wood, and other toys with sharp edges, wrap tender spots with sports wrap or self-clinging bandages or pad the irritating parts of the toy.

Circulation Issues

When the restraints are too tight and the bottom's skin color changes to unnatural shades of red, purple, yellow, white, or blue, or the skin becomes unnaturally cold and clammy, there's likely a serious problem with circulation. Don't wait. Immediately loosen the restraint, adjust the bondage, or change position.

Nerve compression

It's the "pins and needles" sensation. There's no way for the top to know this is happening, as there's no color or temperature change to the skin. The only way they'll know is if the bottom reports it. Bottoms—report it! Don't ignore slight sensations of tingling. It could be an early warning of a serious problem. I almost lost the use of my left hand when I was first exploring bondage because I disregarded a persistent tingling during a lovely long scene.

Allergies (latex, nickel and other metals, natural rope fiber, leather treatments, etc.)

If you know you're allergic to certain materials, avoid them. If you develop a rash, itchiness, swelling, or trouble breathing every time you play with a certain toy, you're likely allergic to the material. Some medications can cause allergy-like reactions to certain materials as well. Consult your physician or get tested for allergies. Let your play partner know of any allergies or other conditions.

Breathing Issues
The ability to breathe is really popular. Everyone loves to do it on a regular, ongoing basis and it's key to not dying in bondage. Make sure to keep the bottom's breathing unobstructed. If he's congested, don't use a big ball gag or close off his mouth in any way. Don't use a hood that closes his nose and then insert a gag, push his face into a pillow, or shove a large hard body part down his throat. Don't wrap the entire head with cling wrap, obstructing both the nose and mouth. Yes, these examples are all from true bondage accidents.

Neck Issues
Along with not obstructing the bottom's ability to breathe, take care not to damage the larynx. Don't tighten the bondage around the neck in such a way that the front of the neck is crushed. Don't use a dog collar and pull the leash hard from behind. Don't use the neck as one end of a predicament hogtie against the feet. Again, these instances were all reported in real bondage tragedies.

MY LITTLE SEX SLAVE

Ingredients
locking collar
leash
leather wrist restraints with connector clips
leather ankle restraints with connector clips
your favorite sex toys, lube, safer sex supplies, and whatever else you enjoy in your usual sex life

Action
Read Chapter 3, How to Train Your Sex Slave, by Laura Antoniou, and Chapter 11, Stop, Drop, and Role! Erotic Role Playing, by Mollena Williams. Study up on these practices.

Install bondage attachment points on your bed in advance.

Agree that the collar symbolizes belonging and service. You may choose to agree to special names during this scene.

With gravity and adoration, put the collar on the bottom and lock it. Put the key within reach in a safe place.

Apply wrist restraints and connect them.

Apply ankle restraints and connect them.

Rotate the D-ring of the collar to the front of the neck and clip the leash on.

Commence sexing!

Use the leash to direct the bottom where you want him.

When you want him in a new position, change the restraint clip arrangement. Unclip all the restraints and connect them to the bed attachment points. Faceup or facedown, which would you prefer?

Sex some more.

Give aftercare deliciously.

OTHER BONDAGE BLOOPERS
Duct Tape
Duct tape and similarly serious adhesive tape are nasty on the skin. They can rip off skin and hair. Some people even get rashes.

Don't Leave the Bottom Alone
A few years ago a hot bondage scene ended in death when the top stepped away to let the bottom enjoy a mummified sensory deprivation scene. Something went wrong while he was gone, and when the top returned he wasn't able to revive his lover. If the bottom can't move well enough to correct problems, don't leave them unattended. If you want to make the bottom think you left the room, that's easy: blindfold the bottom, walk loudly out of the room with your shoes on, remove the shoes, and then tiptoe back into the room.

Hotel-Room Coffee Tables
I'll admit to this one. They're just not as sturdy as they look. It's really hard to find wood glue at 9 a.m., before checkout.

Bathroom
Bottoms, this one's for you. Go to the bathroom before the fun starts!

What's most important is that you and your partners have fun. As I say in my classes, "Don't kill 'em, don't harm 'em, don't bore 'em." As long as the mutual communication is clear and basic safety is attended to, don't stress out about doing something wrong. Bondage is a form of pleasure art where, once you know the basics, the creative potential is endless. Now that you're armed with information and ideas, go forth, explore, and have fabulous bondage sex!

CHAPTER 6

A LITTLE COCK AND BALL PLAY

HARDY HABERMAN

What starts as a playful little diversion can became a supercharged sexual romp with a little imagination and a few toys. I'm talking about a practice commonly called *cock and ball torture*, or CBT. Now, don't let that word *torture* stop you. Most of what we call CBT is playful and fun, and it can be as wild or as tame as you and your partner desire.

A man's genitals are both very sensitive and very resilient. This means they can take a lot of stress as well as be delightfully responsive to sensations both intense and mild. Add to this the emotional investment men have in the equipment between their legs and you get an ideal playground for a creative partner with a kinky streak.

Before trying any kind of CBT, it's important to establish

good communication with your partner. If you are a man playing with another man, you can use your own experience to gauge how sensations might feel for your partner, but remember that everyone experiences sensations differently. Just because you have a penis, you can't assume your partner's penis will react the same way as yours. Communicating about what is working and what is not working is important.

For a woman playing with a man, it's even more essential to keep channels of communication open during the scene. It might not conform to your fantasy of what should happen, but for the first few times it's better to have a good dialogue while the scene is going on. This will make future encounters easier and give you and your partner more confidence. Once you have this experience, adding more elaborate fantasy elements will be easier and more rewarding.

A cock and ball torture scene is something you build up to—not jump into. Now, if that sounds overly cautious, so be it. I never like to play recklessly with my partner's genitals, since I usually want the opportunity to play with them again. Therefore, I err on the side of caution, even when I have confidence in what I am doing. As the person in control of a scene, it's my job to be responsible for my partner's safety and well-being. If you break your toys, you can't play with them again.

Cock and ball torture, or *cock and ball play*, as I think it is more aptly called, requires nothing more than a pair of hands and a good imagination, but a wide variety of toys are made specifically for this kind of fun. Since you may not want to invest a lot of money in toys you might use once and find you don't really like, I suggest the following for a beginner's collection: a coil of braided nylon rope, some wooden clothespins, an elastic bandage (like an ACE bandage), and a toothbrush. With just these few items and your imagination you and your partner can explore almost all the basic sensations in CBT.

Nora had planned a special evening for Bob. They had been dating for many months and spent a lot of time talking about their fantasies, both sexual and otherwise. Bob had expressed an interest in letting Nora take the upper hand in their bedroom play and he told her some vivid stories of what he imagined could happen. She was not only attentive, but enthusiastic. Nora relished the idea of taking a dominant role with Bob during their sex play, so she prepared to make at least a few of his fantasies come true.

"Lock the door," she told him in a breathy voice. She stood waiting for his compliance like a female drill sergeant, hands behind her back.

Bob paused for a second and then snapped into action. He picked up on what was going on and was eager to comply.

"Now, I want you naked before you go any further into my house!"

Bob couldn't undress fast enough. Shedding his clothes with speed, he left them scattered around the entrance hall. When he had finally removed the last garment, his underwear, he stood before her feeling aroused and very vulnerable.

"You will not leave your clothes all over my house. Fold them neatly and bring them with you."

She turned her back and moved away from the door. Bob

did his best gathering up his stuff and at least made an effort to fold it into a single bundle. Then, like an obedient puppy, he followed Nora into the bedroom.

"Where do you want me to put these?"

Nora looked at him standing there naked, his cock already almost completely hard.

"What did you say, boy?" She put a special emphasis on that last word.

Bob took a few seconds to process her question and then it dawned on him.

"Where do you want me to put these, Mistress?"

Nora smiled and pointed to the dresser and tried to stifle a grin. She had never seen Bob so naked and vulnerable. She was almost as excited as he was.

"Now kneel on the bed facing me." Nora pointed to the bed.

Bob scrambled onto the bed and knelt facing his partner. Anticipating what was coming, he spread his legs slightly and held his hands behind his back, giving Nora a full view of and full access to his now fully erect cock.

After a little more dialogue, Nora was satisfied that Bob was ready for the games to begin. She made sure he understood how he was to address her and how he was to let her know how her play was affecting him.

"I will satisfy my desires," Nora said, getting into the mood of the character. "If at any time you feel you can no longer submit to my desires, you will ask for 'mercy.' Do you understand?"

"Yes, Mistress, I will ask for mercy."

COMMUNICATION

CBT can be great fun when combined with a dominant/submissive scene or dynamic. You can incorporate the learning curve into the play while maintaining the power exchange. For example, as the scene progresses, the dominant partner can demand responses from the submissive partner: "Do you like that, boy?" or "Does that make you horny, boy?" Not only does it give both partners a sense of who is in control, but the back-and-forth dialogue lets the submissive give honest feedback.

One word of caution: injuries to the male genitals can result in some serious repercussions. It's a good idea to let the partner on the receiving end have the ultimate say in matters of pain and sensation. A man, even one who is aroused and eager to please his partner, knows when something feels wrong with his genitals, and that means you need a signal that things have progressed beyond tolerable levels. You should always have a safeword. In addition, I like to use this method of communication: I tell my partner that as long as he is having fun he should address me as "Sir," and if we need to talk, he should call me by my real name. That way the flow of communication can keep going without bringing things to a screeching halt.

Once you and your intended playmate have established some method of communication, it's time to get down to business.

Nora began by taking a piece of rope and making several wraps at the base of Bob's penis, looping behind his balls with each wrap. As she wrapped the rope she made sure it was tight enough to be confining but not so tight as to be painful. After three or four wraps, Bob's penis was harder than ever. Then she took the ends of the rope and tied them together. The remaining rope she pulled up and inserted between Bob's teeth.

"Hold that tight, do you hear me?"

Bob answered with a garbled, "Yes, Mistress."

ROPE BONDAGE

It can be more fun than you might imagine to tie up someone's cock; the feeling of taking power from your partner by immobilizing his genitals is hot, and for him, the sensation of having the tight rope around the base of his cock and balls is very erotic. I suggest using a coil of braided nylon rope that is about nine feet long. Take one end of the rope, leaving about a foot of rope free to tie the end. Wrap the rope around the base of the cock several times; loop the rope behind the balls with each wrap. The coils of rope should be tight and coiled closely, as if you are winding it around a spool, to actually stretch the skin of the genitals away from the body. Be careful not to pinch this skin between the coils of rope—that is *not* an erotic experience. After you have about five or six wraps, tie off the rope using the one-foot length and the remaining rope. When done, you should have several feet of rope left (as Nora did in the passage above). Doing this also allows your partner to tighten or loosen the tension on the rope, and that gives him yet another safety valve if the sensations get too intense.

Now that his equipment was nicely held in place, Nora could begin her work in earnest. She retrieved the toothbrush from the nightstand drawer where she had stashed it. Holding it before Bob, she could see the puzzled look in his eyes.

"You know what this is, boy?"

Bob nodded, the puzzled expression starting to fade as he realized what she had in store.

"I am not going to brush your teeth, you know."

Bob understood all too clearly what she was going to do, and as she took hold of his rock-hard penis, he winced at the sensation he expected would be coming soon.

Nora took the toothbrush and slowly rubbed the bristles across the head of Bob's cock. It was a very light brushing sensation, but to a man with an erection, the head of the penis is very, very sensitive.

Bob moaned, giving Nora a sense of perverse pleasure knowing she was not only in control, but able to affect him so much with such little effort. She brushed the head of his dick again, this time even slower and with a little more pressure.

"Ooooweee," *Bob mumbled, still holding the rope obediently between his teeth.*

"Sensitive, boy?" *Nora prodded.*

"Yes, Mistress," *Bob mumbled, letting Nora know he was feeling it but still enjoying the game.*

Nora then brushed around the underside of the head of his cock. Bob stiffened and shook—the sensations were at once irritating and yet enjoyable.

SENSATION IMPLEMENTS

The mildly abrasive touch of a toothbrush can be very intense, especially when used on the head of the penis. Using a soft-bristle model can pretty much ensure that you won't do any damage, but you may also use stiffer bristles if you wish. Though the skin of the penis would seem very delicate, it's actually pretty resilient, and as long as you are careful, you can deliver a lot of stimulation. Be careful not to actually abrade the skin, or cut it. Though your partner will most likely recover, there is always a chance of infection if the skin is broken, so use caution. Other fun toys for this kind of sensation play are paintbrushes, nylon scouring pads, mushroom brushes, feathers, and just about anything that can deliver a variety of sensations. Browsing in your kitchen gadget drawer can produce a bonanza of CBT toys!

Nora took a roll of elastic bandage out of the nightstand drawer. She wrapped the bandage around Bob's scrotum. Starting at the base of his cock, she began stretching the bandage and wrapping it around the flexible skin of his balls. As she wrapped, his testicles were naturally pushed farther away from his body, stretching the normally wrinkled skin over his testicles. When she was finished, the result was interesting to look at. The tight skin of his scrotum now seemed to shine from being pulled taut. His balls were stretched away from his body by almost two inches.

Her final touch was to use the fastener that came with the bandage to secure it to itself, being careful to make sure the hooks didn't pierce the folds of the bandage.

"What a nice package that makes, don't you think so, boy?"

Bob tried to see what she was doing, but his hard cock was in the way. "Yes, Mistress."

Now Nora rubbed the brush over the shiny skin of Bob's bound balls. Bob twitched and jerked at the intense sensations. She was careful not to apply too much pressure, but it still made Bob wince and jerk with every stroke.

As she looked at her handiwork, she noticed a few drops of precum emerging from the head of Bob's cock.

BANDAGE BONDAGE

Using the elastic bandage is a simple skill, and if you have ever bandaged a wrist or ankle, it's pretty much the same thing. Again, maintain communication with your partner and avoid making the wraps too tight. You want to constrain the scrotum, not cut off all blood flow. Also be careful with the metal clip that is used to fasten the bandage, making sure there are sufficient layers of elastic between the teeth of the clip and the skin of your partner's balls. When bound properly, the skin of the scrotum will be stretched and the testes will be cradled in a nice neat wrap, looking like an inverted ice cream cone with two scoops of ice cream.

"Well, since you have been so good, I have another surprise for you," Nora said. Reaching into the drawer, she produced a handful of clothespins. As soon as Bob saw these he stiffened and whimpered, but his cock stood even more rigid than before.

Nora stroked his erect dick and felt along the underside for some loose skin. Even erect, most men have a certain amount of skin that can be used for CBT, and Bob was no exception. She gently pinched the skin on the underside of his shaft, careful not to pinch the urethra, the conduit that carries both urine and sperm through the penis. She pulled some of the skin away from the shaft, and at the base near his balls she attached a clothespin.

Bob whimpered again but said nothing. Taking this as a signal that he was still in the game, Nora continued to add clothespin after clothespin, working her way up the shaft until she came to the head.

Bob was breathing heavily now in short gasps, so Nora asked the question, "Do you like pleasing me this way, boy?"

Trembling Bob replied, "Yes, Mistress, but I'm not sure how much more I can take." Then he added, "Mistress."

"Don't worry, boy, that's all we are going to use for now." She moved closer to him and kissed his chest, running her tongue over his nipples and tracing a circle around his navel. She took her time, letting the clothespins do their work for a while.

CLIPS, CLAMPS, AND OTHER THINGS THAT PINCH

You can use clothespins as well as clips for snack chip bags, hair clips, and just about anything that pinches to create unique sensations. I suggest testing clips on the skin between your thumb and forefinger if you are experimenting. If you can't endure the sensation there, your partner certainly won't be able to endure them on his private parts.

While different types of clamps can produce different sensations, generally when you clamp a section of the flesh of the penis, the body has both a physical and a chemical reaction. The nerve receptors in the skin sense the pain of the clothespins and signal to your brain there is distress. Your brain reacts, as good brains should, by sending out impulses generating adrenaline. This quickens your heart rate, preparing the body for possible danger, even though you know you're in safe hands. You may feel yourself breathing more quickly or your voice may quaver.

Additionally, the brain signals the body to produce some natural opiates to relieve the pain. It usually takes longer for these to respond, so the painful sensations persist for a while.

The clothespins also cut off some circulation to the nerve receptors in your skin, and after a few minutes the receptors go numb and the pain sensation subsides, leaving you possibly still quivering but able to tolerate the sensations of the clothespins. The Top should continue to check in with his or her partner to make sure that the sensations are not simply painful but also erotic. As a rule of thumb, don't leave the clips on more than 10 minutes for starters. Long periods of compression can cause nerve damage, and though it is rare, again, I urge caution. Perhaps surprisingly, once the sensation of pain has numbed, leaving the clips on longer has little effect.

When clamps or clothespins are removed, the blood rushes back into the skin and reawakens the nerve receptors; the receptors fire off their distress message to the brain with renewed vigor, and the bottom usually experiences intense pain.

Nora looked at the row of clothespins and couldn't resist toying with them. This action made Bob jump as new sensations delivered their messages to his brain.

Nora caressed his hard cock and leaned down to lick the head. She looked up at Bob, who trembled more than before. The sight of her luscious lips nibbling at his dick and the new sensations of pain and pleasure were working to make this a memorable night.

Nora took the head of his cock into her mouth, careful not to disturb the pins. She used her tongue to stimulate the underside of his head, right where she had used the cruel toothbrush just minutes before. She figured he deserved a little reward for being so obedient, and besides, she loved the feeling of his cock in her mouth.

While she lovingly sucked the head of his cock, she used her fingers to flick the clothespins. Her long nails scraping against the row of pins sent flashes of pain through Bob's cock. She waited a bit and then did it again, each time making Bob twitch and squirm. His moaning was intoxicating to her, knowing she was giving him a wonderfully twisted delight of pain and pleasure together.

Removing her mouth from his head, she lifted his dick almost up to his belly, the clothespins protruding toward her face. This time, as she looked up at him, she had a slightly evil grin. She opened her mouth and, using her teeth, delicately took the uppermost clothespin in her mouth.

The sensation was like white-hot lead coursing through his body. Bob grimaced. "Motherfucker," he said, almost dropping the rope.

"Motherfucker, who?" Nora demanded.

"Motherfucker, Mistress?"

"Much better, boy," she said, chuckling as she approached the next pin. Each one she removed with care so as not to damage the delicate skin of Bob's penis. Each one brought a new invective from Bob, followed by a polite "Mistress," right up to the last one.

"Mercy, Mistress," Bob panted, feeling as if he could take no more.

"Unfortunately," Nora said, "that clothespin has to come off and it's going to hurt, so why don't I let you take it off?"

Bob thought for a moment and then closed his eyes tight. "No, Mistress, go ahead."

"Go ahead, what?" she questioned. "Have you forgotten your manners?"

"Please, Mistress, take it off."

She smiled and bent down, taking the final pin between her teeth. She slowly squeezed the pin, releasing the tension and letting the last bit of skin pull free.

For a moment Bob didn't make a sound. Then he began giggling uncontrollably. The combination of adrenaline and natural opiates had him higher than a kite.

"Thank you, Mistress."

Nora slowly unwrapped his balls from the bandage and reached up to remove the rope from his mouth. Untying it, she carefully removed the coil of rope, making sure not to pull too much hair in the process.

Once free, Bob's cock was still erect. Nora intended to make good use of it over the course of the night. Now it was time for his reward. Both Nora and Bob knew it would be a scene they would enjoy again, but now it was time for just plain lust.

CHAPTER 7

KINKY TWISTED TANTRA

BARBARA CARRELLAS

The place on the erotic map where the paths of Tantric sex and BDSM intersect was once as lonely and obscure as a tiny no-pub town in the Australian outback. Not only was it nearly impossible to find, hardly anyone looked for it because no one believed it actually existed. In recent years things have changed dramatically. Some Tantric practitioners are now combining elements of power and intense sensation with traditional Tantra in a variation sometimes referred to as Dark Tantra. Longtime BDSM players are coming out of the closet as spiritual seekers and creating scenes intentionally designed to welcome god/goddess/universe/all-that-is into the dungeon. Communities in which kinky people and Tantrikas meet, mingle, and play together are growing and now can be found all over the world.

It's not surprising that it's taken a while for these two communities to find common ground. From a stylistic point of view, it would appear that people wearing leather and wielding floggers would have little or nothing in common with people wearing sarongs and stroking each other with feathers. But like most everything else in life, outward appearances and preconceived notions have little or nothing to do with the essence of an erotic or spiritual art form.

Tantric sex and BDSM have much more in common than may seem apparent at first glance. Both are erotic arts of consciousness. Both arts add intensity to life and sex. Both embrace a wide variety of powerful consensual practices. Both Tantric and BDSM rituals are about raising erotic energy. Both practices involve conscious giving and receiving. Both encourage risks—either physical or emotional. Both erotic arts encourage personal freedom, individuality, and imagination. And both produce trance states, and transcendental, transformational experiences.

Why has it taken this long for BDSM aficionados and Tantrikas to discover each other's charms? One of the stumbling blocks has been the lack of a common language. The two communities have traditionally described what, how, and why they do what they do in language that has sounded off-putting, inflated, or obscure to anyone not in the club. One of the primary missions of my work has been to translate words, actions, and intentions across sexual boundaries. So before we go any further, let's define some terms.

WHAT IS TANTRA?

Tantra is the ancient Eastern spiritual practice that embraces sex as a legitimate and effective path to enlightenment. Tantra is an embodied spiritual practice. It embraces all elements and aspects of life—including but not limited to sex—as a way to experience direct knowledge of the divine. Notice I call it a spiritual practice, not a religion. Religions tend to approach spirituality in a controlled, ordered manner. There is usually a hierarchical organization and an emphasis upon a particular set of rules. If you follow the rules, you are promised a predictable goal of salvation or enlightenment or peace.

Can you have a wild, ecstatic, spiritual experience within a religion? Absolutely. You can have a wild, ecstatic, spiritual experience within the context of almost anything. For many of us, however, spiritual experiences are easier to create within the context of a spiritual practice. A spiritual practice is just that: practice. You consistently practice a way of being and seeing in the world that invites the unknown, the unexpected, and the chaotic. Spiritual practices encourage you to step out of your ordinary reality into a realm of infinite possibilities where you are likely to find that there is no separation between you and everything else, including god—goddess—universe—divine—all that-is.

What Is Consciousness?

Tantrically speaking, being conscious simply means that you are in a relaxed state of awareness with a quiet mind able to focus gently and easily on what's going on in the present moment. It's mindfulness. It's putting your attention on your intentions. To be conscious is to go totally into whatever you are doing—whatever it is you are experiencing. When I talk about conscious sex, I am talking about a sexual encounter in which you are focused on each successive moment of your journey through pleasure. It is not a goal-oriented activity. In Tantric sex not even orgasm can be a goal, because there is no goal. Orgasms certainly do happen—all the time, in fact. But you are likely to find other erotic moments as exquisite as orgasm on this goal-free path.

What Is Tantric Sex?

Tantric sex is a way to explore and experience sex that includes and encourages a spiritual experience. Tantra (and Taoist sexuality, which started as a branch of Chinese medicine) sees sex as an energy rather than an activity. In Tantra we use techniques such as breath, touch, sound, and movement to move the sexual energy that starts in the genitals into the rest of the body, effectively turning the entire body into a sex organ. During sex with a partner, we build and exchange this energy with a beloved. Consciousness plays a vital role in this exchange, because as you increase your level of consciousness, you increase the intensity of the energy within yourself and between the two of you.

TANTRIC SEX TECHNIQUES

There is an entire universe of possibilities to be discovered when we blend Tantra's focus on energy, consciousness, and spiritual connection with BDSM's traditions of consent, negotiation, and intensity. In order to experience the deep erotic sensations that can carry us into prolonged ecstatic states of arousal and altered states of consciousness, we first have to slow down and get back to basics. In that sentence we find the first of these basics: *Slow down!* In Tantra, we do not slow down just for the sake of making sex last longer. Rather, slowing down is the natural consequence of being more conscious. So as you practice the following basics, remember that it's not about how fast or how intensely you practice, but how much consciousness you bring to your practice.

We're going to begin by focusing on the physical, nongenital components of a great sexual experience. Nongenital? Aren't genitals the most important part of sex? Well, no. In fact, you can have amazing, prolonged, full-body orgasms by combining the following nongenital techniques. And these basic elements are not just essential in the practice of Tantra—they are actually the building blocks of all erotic experiences. So let's take a deep breath, drop into our bodies, and discover all the ways that we can generate, enjoy, and share massive amounts of sexual energy.

Breathe

Our breath is our greatest source of energy and aliveness, yet most of us breathe just enough to stay alive. If you are not already a dedicated erotic breathwork junkie, I strongly suggest you become one. Deep, full conscious breathing can take you higher and deeper and farther than any other sex toy or technique. Regrettably, instead of breathing more, most of us tend to *stop* breathing in intensely erotic situations. I attribute this to a rule that almost all of us learned as adolescents. I call it the Quiet and Quick Rule. When we were first masturbating on a regular basis, we had to be quiet so that other members of the family would not hear us. We had to be quick so that we could get to orgasm before we were discovered. How did we manage to be quiet and quick? We held our breath. There was no chance of accidentally making a sound if you weren't breathing. Unfortunately, the constant repetition of the Quiet and Quick Rule imprinted in it on our muscle memory, in much the same way that we learned to type or ride a bicycle. So now when we approach orgasm or any other peak erotic experience, we tend to hold our breath. To reach the level of erotic heights we long for, and to get the most out of the commingling of Tantra and BDSM, we need to break this habit and reprogram our bodies with breath.

There are many different breath techniques that can bring you to a great variety of ecstatic states. But all you really need to know is this: breathing in and out through your nose is relaxing, particularly when you make the exhale longer than the inhale. Breathing in and out through your mouth is energizing. You can alternate the two to produce states of relaxed, alive awareness. The most important thing to remember is to *just keep breathing*. If all you do is keep breathing a bit more fully and deeply than you usually do, you'll be well on your way to a delightfully altered state of consciousness.

Begin by practicing on your own. As you masturbate, breathe in and out through your mouth fully and deeply. Keep your throat and mouth relaxed, and don't force the exhale. If conscious breathing is new to you, you'll inevitably find that you go back to holding your breath. Don't criticize yourself, just bring your attention back to your breath. You'll probably notice that it takes you a bit longer to orgasm when you're breathing like this. Imagine your body as 30-gallon container waiting to be filled with erotic energy. When you hold your breath while trying to orgasm, you are only able to generate enough energy to fill up an area around your genitals about the size of a coffee cup. When you breathe fully and consistently for longer, you generate enough energy to fill your entire 30-gallon tank. Now, which container of fuel would you rather have to power your orgasm? Breathe.

Give Your Mind Erotically Constructive Things to Do
Our minds wander. They jump from thought to thought. It's not a bad thing; it's just what minds do. If we don't deliberately keep our attention on the erotic present moment, our minds will dance us right out of the room into some mundane anxiety, or into a fantasy that takes us out of our body and away from what's actually happening right here, right now.

One of the most effective ways of seducing our minds into becoming our erotic allies is to focus on the creation and movement of erotic energy. This is not as difficult or as boring as it may sound. For example, if you are flogging someone, you might imagine erotic energy pumping up from your genitals into your heart, through your arm, out the tips of your flogger, and into your partner's heart. When your partner exhales, you can imagine their erotic energy flying out of their heart and coming back to you.

With some practice you will actually be able to see energy running through other people's bodies and feel it running through yours. For example, if you are the one being flogged, you can imagine your heart being cracked open with each stroke. Or you can imagine the fiery strokes of a cane lighting your own inner fire and burning away limitations.

As with the breathing, practice by yourself first. As you masturbate, imagine breathing the turn-on in your genitals up into your heart, then into the top of your head. Feel it sliding into your arms and hands, legs and feet. You might feel the energy move, or see it, or even hear it. It doesn't matter which way you imagine it. And feel free to fake it until you feel it. Energy follows thought. When you pretend the energy is in your heart or your hands, chances are you'll be feeling it there soon after.

In both sex and BDSM we can become overly concerned with technique. We worry that we're not doing it as well as it should be done, or as well as it could be done, or as well as it was done by our lover's last partner. If you focus on breath and energy, there will be a lot less room in your mind for this kind of self-criticism. And, if you follow the energy instead of your critical mind, you won't have to figure out what to do next. You'll already be doing it.

Play at the Resilient Edge of Resistance
This is not really a technique. It's a magical piece of awareness, crystallized and named by my beloved late teaching partner, Chester Mainard. As with most energetic practices, it is very

simple but it may take a little practice before it becomes easy, natural, and automatic.

Although the Resilient Edge of Resistance applies to any kind of connection, especially emotional and psychic connections, it is most easily understood when applied to touch. The Resilient Edge of Resistance is a touch that is neither too hard nor too soft. The touch is deep enough that the body pushes back just a little, but gentle enough that the body does not go rigid. When you are touched at your Resilient Edge of Resistance you are lulled into a place of deep comfort and surrender, yet you remain awake and eager for more.

Try it on your arm or leg. First try a touch that's too gentle and soft. Feel how it's kind of creepy and annoying? Now try a touch that's too hard. Feel how the body tries to pull away, or goes rigid to defend itself? Now find the place—it will feel like a kind of holding—where the touch is just right. Begin to massage your arm or your leg. As you continue the massage, notice how your touch changes. As the body relaxes, you can go a little deeper.

The Resilient Edge of Resistance applies to all kinds of touch including the kind of intense sensation that happens in some BDSM play. We all know that we can't start off using our heaviest toy with our greatest strength without burning out our bottom in two strokes. We start with warm-up strokes, staying at the bottom's Resilient Edge of Resistance, gradually building up the intensity, until we're both flying happily on the exquisitely extreme sensation.

Play with Sound

Sounds of pleasure can be embarrassing or frightening for some people. Remember the Quiet and Quick Rule? We learn at an early age not to make too much noise while having sex. However, sound moves energy—a lot of energy. Whether you are enjoying a long delicious fuck or a long intense night in the dungeon, you'll get a lot more turned on and reach higher ecstatic states if you make some noise. In Tantra, the body's energetic anatomy is made up of chakras—spinning spirals of energy located in approximately the same areas as the glands of the endocrine system—at the perineum, lower belly, solar plexus, heart, throat, forehead (aka third eye), and crown. Each of these seven chakras has a sound associated with it (as well as specific physical and metaphysical qualities, colors, and symbols). The first chakra has the lowest pitch, the highest chakra the highest pitch. You can move energy up and down your body by making sounds of different pitches. You don't have to know any Sanskrit chants—all you have to do is remember to make sounds

Use PC Squeezes

PC squeezes, also known as Kegels, are little squeezes of the pubococcygeus muscle. The PC muscle is the muscle you use to stop the flow of urine. Find your PC muscle now and give it a little squeeze. Your PC muscle is your own personal erotic energy pump. Think of it as a heat pump on the furnace in your erotic basement. Use PC squeezes to help you get turned on, then to move your turn-on up through your body and out into your arms and legs. Without your PC heat pump, sexual energy might eventually get into all the rooms of your house, but with PC squeezes it will get there so much faster and more effectively.

Create Connection with Eye-Gazing

The Tantric technique of eye-gazing is at once challenging, intimate, and a trust exercise of the highest order. It is also mesmerizing, erotically hypnotizing, and deeply comforting. Tantrikas believe that prolonged eye-gazing gives you a glimpse into your partner's soul. At the very least, eye-gazing and breathing together will create a deep connection. Different Tantric traditions have different opinions about which eye to gaze into and why, but it really doesn't matter. I like to gaze into my partner's eyes with relaxed, softly focused eyes. However, in a scene involving power exchange, my gaze would likely turn more direct and commanding.

Safe, Sane, and Consensual/Risk-Aware Consensual Kink

Traditionally, the six ways to generate and circulate sexual energy described above have been considered Tantric techniques. "Safe, sane, and consensual" (SSC) and "risk-aware consensual kink" (RACK) have been considered exclusively BDSM principles. Agreeing to take proper safety precautions, connect in a sober and conscious state of mind, and play consensually is excellent advice for anyone engaged in any sort of erotic play. From an energetic point of view, these principles create a safe enclosure where we are able to take the kinds of emotional risks that are necessary to fly in intimate connection with others and within ourselves. They are, if you will, the magic carpet on which we ride.

Now that you've got the basics, let's practice some kinky twisted Tantra, or if you prefer, Tantric BDSM. We'll do this by looking at two of the most basic components of BDSM—Power and Pain—through a Tantric lens.

D/s Tantra: Power
There is virtually no human interaction that does not involve some exchange of power. Because BDSM is a consensual erotic art form, the power exchange we play with is power *sharing with* someone, not power *over* someone. So long as the safe, sane, and consensual rule is in play, our power is on loan, never taken away by force. The roles in power exchange might be named dominant/submissive, top/bottom, or any number of other more personalized descriptions of this temporary binary. Whatever the labels, both partners are regarded as equally powerful. After all, you have to have some power in order to be able to gift it to someone for a while.

There is an equivalent dynamic in Tantra, where the labels are more likely to be yin/yang or masculine/feminine. In Tantra all genders are considered equally powerful. The energetic principles of *consciousness* and *energy* are represented by the god Shiva and the goddess Shakti, respectively. As legend has it, when Shiva joined in sexual union with Shakti the union of pure consciousness and pure energy gave birth to the world. Obviously, everyone has aspects of both consciousness and energy, just as everyone has both masculine and feminine qualities. In some branches of neo-Tantra these energetic principles were mistakenly reduced to the binaries of male and female. This created not only a gender bias but also a heterosexist bias. In Tantric circles today, this misconception is now much less prevalent than it once was.

We all have our issues around power and gender. As the daughter of a mother with borderline personality disorder, I lived in a nonconsensual D/s relationship for the first 18 years of my life. As such, I have had a lifelong uneasy relationship with power exchange—even conscious, consensual, power exchange. As a radical queer (I describe myself most frequently as a young black drag queen in a blonde female body), I have had an uneasy relationship with the masculine/feminine binary. My sensitivity to being boxed into any of these roles meant I had to reinvent them to be able to find my own path in both Tantra and BDSM. I needed to find new language—language that did not stir up old traumas.

I looked for words that described the essence of the energy exchange, not the identity of the participants. I have tried giver/receiver, creative/receptive, initiator/beneficiary. The words that work best for me? Active and receptive.

For me, active and receptive are like positive and negative poles on a battery. One pole is not better or stronger than the other. You need both to create energy. In practice, assuming active and receptive roles is a delightful, efficient way of amping up energy. Once the energy is firing on its own, the roles begin to slip away, becoming unnecessary and even meaningless—as both active and receptive partners are carried along on currents of flowing energy.

EXERCISE: PLAYING WITH POWER

Let's try an erotic exercise in which you can experience the essence of active and receptive power exchange.

This exercise will require a partner, a blindfold, and wrist restraints. If you don't have a pair of wrist cuffs you can make wrist restraints out of a 15- to 18-foot piece of rope. Choose ¼-inch to ½-inch-thick soft rope. Although this is not a bondage exercise, you will need to know how to tie wrist restraints safely without damaging nerves or cutting off circulation. Instructions for simple wrist bondage follow below.

One of you will be the active partner, the other the receptive partner. Read through these instructions in advance, so you can raise any issues of consent that need to be discussed in the first moments of the exercise.

Playing with Power—Part One

Both partners: Face your partner. Breathe. Gaze into your partner's eyes. Drop into the present moment.

If you have any limits or boundaries around anything in this exercise, share them with your partner now.

Place your right hand on your partner's heart. Then place your left hand over your partner's right hand, which is on your heart. Continue breathing together and eye-gazing. Let this continue until you feel that you have created a deep connection.

Active partner:
1. Fold your rope in half. The loop created where the rope folds is called the bight. Have your partner hold their wrists parallel to each other with their palms facing each other. Make sure the wrists are not touching each other or you won't be able to finish the restraints. Wrap the folded rope around your partner's wrists three or four times.
2. Cross the ends of the rope.
3. Pull the ends to create a twist.

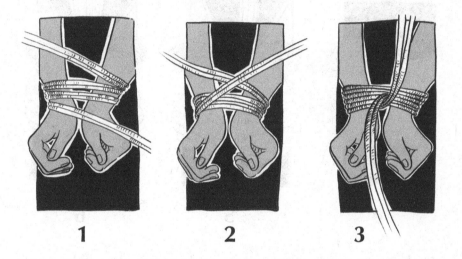

Illustration 7.1. Simple rope handcuffs

Continued on p. 154.

4. Now drop both the bight and the ends between the wrists on either side of the wrapped rope.
5. Bring the bight and the ends back up between the wrists, wrapping around the existing rope, creating rope handcuffs. Don't make the cuffs too tight. You should be able to fit one or two fingers between the bondage and the skin.
6. Tie it off with a simple square knot. You should have enough rope dangling free to use as leash.

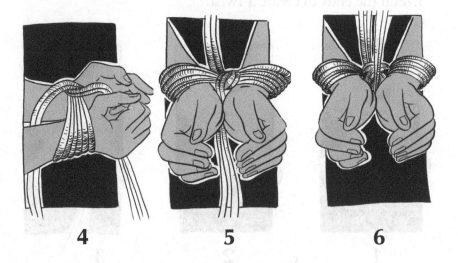

Both partners: Return to eye-gazing. Breathe with your partner. The wrist restraints will have changed the dynamic between you—simply notice how. With your breath and your eyes, begin to take on your active or your receptive role. There is no right or wrong way to do this, nor will the change happen all at once. Just breathe and eye-gaze with the intention of becoming more active or more receptive.

Active partner: Now put the blindfold over your partner's eyes. In a moment you will begin to lead your partner around the room. But before you begin to walk, synchronize your breathing to your partner's. Because you are the active partner, you get to choose the nature of the breath. You can stand behind your partner with your chest against their back, placing your hand on their heart and breathing, making clear your intention that they match their breath to yours. As you begin to walk, this breath can act as the secondary leash between you.

Slowly begin to walk your partner around the room, leading them with the leash. As you lead them, go more completely into the active role. What is demanded from you in this role? Your partner is blindfolded and their hands are tied. This makes you completely responsible for their physical and emotional safety. What energetic techniques can you bring into play to make you as conscious as possible in this moment?

Receptive partner: With each breath, give over a little more control to your active partner. Observe your feelings, as if from a distance. Are you feeling fear? Relief? Resistance? Peace? Although your partner may have established initial control by insisting you match your breath to theirs, as you move into the exercise, experiment with your breath until you find one that helps you move more deeply into receptivity. Remember, a receptive partner is not a passive partner. You are not giving up, giving in, or doing nothing. Rather, you are striving to open up and become more mindful. In this receptive state you are open not only to a more intimate connection with your partner, but to a more intimate connection to yourself, to your surroundings and to all-that-is.

For purposes of this exercise, I strongly suggest you switch roles. You may be involved in a D/s relationship where switching just isn't part of your play. However, that doesn't have to prevent you from experimenting with active and receptive. My friend and colleague Raven Kaldera and his full-time slave, Joshua, figured out a way to experience both active and receptive roles. As Raven described it: "When I was leading Joshua, he was doing what I wanted him to do; when Joshua was leading me, he was doing what he knew I would want him to do."

Playing with Power—Part Two

Now let's experiment with combining power exchange with Tantric positions designed for sexual energy exchange. In order to do this part of the exercise, you'll need to know one energizing breath and one Tantric position. Here's the breath. I call it the Heart Breath:

1. Yawn. Feel how the yawn opens the back of your throat and stretches out your whole mouth and face? That's the feeling of openness you want when you do the Heart Breath.

2. Breathe. Let your mouth fall open slightly. Relax your jaw and face, open the back of your throat, and breathe in through your mouth, gently but fully.

3. Exhale. Don't push the breath out; just let it fall out with a gentle little sigh, *ahhh*.

4. Take in as much air as you can, as effortlessly as you can, then let it go.

5. Keep breathing. That's all there is to it. You can do the Heart Breath as slowly or as intensely as you like.

Now the position. It is called Yab Yum, and it's the classic Tantric sex position. One partner sits in an easy cross-legged posture, with a cushion under their tailbone. The other partner sits in their lap, facing them, with legs wrapped around their waist and the soles of the feet touching. Both partners place their right hand at the back of their partner's neck and their left hand on their partner's tailbone. Yab Yum can be done with or without penetration. For purposes of this exercise, we'll do it without penetration, so you can keep your focus on the power exchange. In Yab Yum you are perfectly aligned with your partner, energetically. You can gaze into your partner's eyes. You can kiss. Or, touch your foreheads together, third eye to third eye. You can draw energy up your partner's spine, from the tailbone to the neck. As you get more and more turned on and active, you can rock back and forth passionately.

Now you're ready to begin part two of the exercise.

Active partner: Lead your partner over to a soft and comfortable but firm and supported place. Beds are generally too soft. Try some soft pillows placed on the floor. Remove the wrist restraints.

Both partners: You are going to begin with an even power exchange, then move into active and receptive roles.

Sit facing your partner in an easy cross-legged position. (If this is difficult for you, arrange some pillows on the floor or sit with your legs in some other more comfortable position.) Place your right hand over your partner's heart. Then place your left hand over your partner's hand, which is on your heart. Breathe together using the Heart Breath and look into each other's eyes. Allow a sigh or *ahhh* to come out every four or five breaths or so. Begin to rock back and forth, focusing on an evenly balanced exchange of energy. Neither of you is intentionally active or receptive. As the rocking becomes faster and more intense, take your hands off each other's hearts and hold them together between you in a prayer position, joining all four

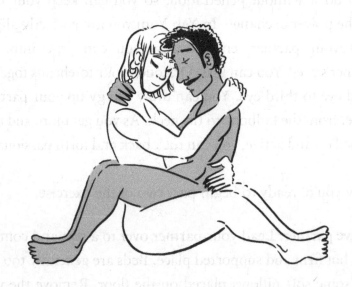

Illustration 7.2. Yab Yum

hands between you. As you rock, move your joined hands in circles—sending energy up the front of your body and down the front of your partner's. Then reverse, sending energy up the front of your partner's body and down the front of yours.

Now, move into Yab Yum. The receptive partner sits in the lap of the active partner. You can breathe with foreheads touching, still eye-gazing, as the active partner begins to rock back and forth. Breathe together with the intention of going *completely and totally* into active and *completely and totally* into receptive.

A variation on this is to tie a (strong) sarong, knotted in the front at the breastbone, on the receptive partner. This gives the active partner a "handle" at the heart chakra. The active partner can "throw" the receptive partner away from them, then pull them back in, building intense energy between the two of you. (Warning: If you choose this variation make sure that the receptive partner's neck and back are flexible enough to withstand the throw. Whiplash is seldom sexy.)

Be aware that odd things can happen during this exercise. The active partner may feel as if they have grown an energetic cock. The receptive partner may feel as if they are being fucked by that cock. Faces can appear to change. You may feel as if you are flying. You may see visions. You may simply enjoy the physical sensation of being thrown about by your partner. You will find your own authentic ecstasy by simple conscious experience of this exercise.

When you have landed safely back on earth, take a moment to analyze the results of your experiment. How did things change when you consciously moved from a balanced power

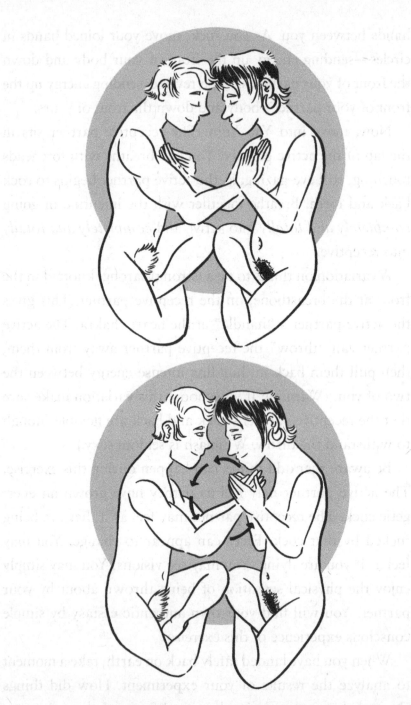

Illustration 7.3. Heart energy exchange

exchange into active and receptive roles? What was that like for you? What was easy? What was hard? Was this type of power exchange different from the ways in which you may have played with power before? As you share the answers to these questions with your partner you will be well on your way to creating your own personalized style of power sharing.

CONSCIOUS SEX

Now that you've had a taste of conscious active and receptive power exchange, let's add conscious sex. Some people get so high off the exchange of power and sexual energy that genital sex becomes irrelevant or redundant. They may intentionally avoid genital orgasm to prolong the ride. However, in addition to feeling wonderful and just being fabulous fun, sex is an important energy builder in its own right. How you combine power exchange and sex is completely up to you. In the Yab Yum position, you can use a penis, a dildo, a double dildo or an anal plug for vaginal or anal penetration. Whether your cock is anatomical or strap-on, the combination of the power exchange, the rocking, and the penetration will exponentially intensify all sensations. Vary the speed of your fucking. Fuck really hard and fast. Then just stop. Do nothing. Let the energy run through you for as long as it can. Maintain your active/receptive power exchange even when you are perfectly still. Then fuck really fast again. You can do a variation on this from the rear. In this position, you can play with your partner's clitoris or cock as you fuck.

You can also use conscious power exchange to enhance

erotic massage. If you are the active partner you can use sensual touch—your hands or your whole body—to communicate the transfer of control. For example your hands on their back might convey the message, "You are my property," or, you might lie on top of your partner, using your weight to take command. You can dictate the pace of your partner's arousal, driving them wild by denying them an orgasm or by insisting on multiple "forced" orgasms. By the way, although it might seem logical that the person giving the massage would be the active partner and the person receiving the massage would be the receptive partner, this is not the only viable power-sharing configuration. The person receiving the massage could be the active partner, directing the receptive partner in giving them exactly the right touch, exactly when they want it.

Power exchange and oral sex are a similarly good mix. As the active partner you could take control of your partner's cock or pussy with your mouth, teasing mercilessly, allowing orgasm only on your terms, in your own time. If you like vampire fantasies, you could imagine feeding on your partner by sucking out their power and their pleasure with your mouth. As the receptive partner, your mouth could become your partner's sex toy, to be used as they please.

Use your imagination. You don't need specifically Tantric positions or BDSM rituals to play with conscious power exchange. Some fantasy or image may have flashed through your mind as you were exchanging power. You may have caught a glimpse of a scene you'd like to act out. Perhaps your inner hapless victim wants to be overpowered by your partner's inner evil villain? Whatever your sexual preferences or desires, you can combine them with power exchange. The possibilities are infinite.

THE TAO OF PAIN

People who love to play with pain do it for a variety of reasons. For many people, traveling on the intense sensation commonly referred to as pain produces altered and expanded states of consciousness. For others, playing with "good" pain alleviates physical, emotional, and psychic "bad" pain. Many people who love "good" pain—meaning conscious pain—experience it as orgasmic, including those who consciously and compassionately inflict the pain upon themselves; for example, solo SM artists and cutters.

Conscious pain is not the kind of pain we experience when we stub our toe or bang our elbow on a door frame. Conscious pain is not accidental, nor is it violent. Orgasmic pain is an intense sensation, received by choice by someone who knows how to turn it into pleasure, relief, or empowerment. It is delivered by someone who knows how to deliver it in measured doses, at the right intervals and intensities.

But still, pain as orgasm? Let's consider for a moment: what exactly is an orgasm? The most common definition might be "a sexual climax attained by stimulation of the genitals and other erogenous zones." That seems incomplete. Perhaps we could add "accompanied by a release of accumulated tension and energy." That's better, but it's nowhere near inclusive enough to contain the kinds of expanded orgasms we want to talk about when we combine Tantra and BDSM. Let's try this:

"An orgasm is a release of tension and expansion of energy flowing through the body/mind and connecting us to spirit."

According to this definition, conscious pain could certainly produce an orgasm. And how you actually do that is simple: you use all the techniques for moving sexual energy through the body that you learned at the beginning of this chapter. If you combine conscious breathing, focused imagination, sounds, and PC squeezes, you could have an orgasm with no genital stimulation whatsoever. Yes—an actual orgasm. I recently proved that this type of hands-free, breath-and-energy orgasm is an actual orgasm by having one inside an fMRI machine. Just as you can add these techniques to sex to produce hugely expanded genital orgasms, you can combine them with pain to produce exquisite paingasms. Of course, this doesn't mean you have to leave out the sex. A combined energy/pain/genital orgasm is truly (and almost literally) a mind-blowing experience. You can use all these techniques of expanded orgasm to keep ecstasy flying through you or you flying through it.

EXERCISE: PLAYING WITH PAIN

So let's try another two-part exercise. We'll explore the possibilities of conscious pain in solo practice first and then with a partner.

Before we begin, here's a word of caution and an alert to a possible trigger: The solo practice of pain, like the solo practice of sex (masturbation) may come attached to feelings of shame, guilt, and self-recrimination. For example, some people feel they're mad or bad because they cut, scratch, pull out hair, or bang their wrists. In this next exercise, I'm going to ask you to drop any self-judgment and focus instead on experiencing the sensation of pain. If that's too difficult for you, or if it triggers bad feelings about yourself, then skip the solo part of this exercise and, if possible, go on to Playing with Pain (For Two).

Playing with Pain (for One)
Get comfortable. Make sure you feel physically and psychically safe. Pain (and sex and most everything else) is seldom ecstatic in unsafe space. Breathe gently but fully, in and out of slightly parted, relaxed lips. With each exhale, imagine all the tension leaving your body through the top of your head and the base of your spine. Squeeze your PC muscle and begin to find the beginning of a turn-on in your genitals. Breathe into that turn-on and imagine it flowing through your whole body, and out into your fingertips and toes.

You are going to practice giving, receiving, and fully experiencing a sensation of pain that you give to yourself.

Find a way to give yourself a stinging or thudding sensation—one that doesn't damage your body. We want to focus on sensation, not injury. You can give yourself a slap, a pinch, a bite, or use your fingernails on any place on your body you can reach. For those of you who are more experienced with pain, you can use a favorite toy from your collection of sensation-producing devices. If you don't have a collection of toys, you can use your hands, mouth, a wooden spoon, or some other implement you can find in your kitchen.

You will give yourself a single sensation. This can mean three slaps, or several seconds of a bite. Sometimes a single, effective, painful sensation can only be created with multiple strokes, therefore those multiple strokes count as a single sensation. You're going to create a single sensation and then dive into that sensation as totally as you can, using your breath, your mind, sound, and PC squeezes to expand the sensation and carry it through your body.

So let's try it. Breathe. Center yourself. Focus. Give yourself the sensation. Now go completely into it. Become the pain. Ride it as a surfer rides a wave—all the way into the beach until it disappears.

Breathe. Do it again. Deliver each stroke at your Resilient Edge of Resistance—right at the place where the pain is enough to make you gasp, but not so intense that you withdraw from it completely.

Playing with Pain (for Two)
Now we are going to try a similar exercise with a partner. The receptive partner will ask the active partner for a single sensation and tell the active partner a) how intense the sensation should be, b) how long the sensation should continue, and c) where on the body they wish to receive it. They will also create a safeword. (Most people play with safewords. Some don't. In this exercise, a safeword is part of the mindfulness of our giving and receiving, so we will use one.)

Let's try it: Face your partner. Breathe. Gaze into your partner's eyes. Drop into the present moment. If you have any physical or emotional limits or boundaries concerning anything in this exercise, share them with your partner now.

The **receptive partner** asks for a sensation. The **active partner** decides whether or not this sensation is something they are willing and able to give. If they are willing to give the requested sensation, they do so. Then they do nothing. They breathe and pause, allowing the receptive partner to fully experience the sensation. When the receptive partner is ready for another sensation they ask for it, perhaps specifying that the next sensation be lighter or harder or something completely different. The role of the active partner is to give the sensation and support the receptive partner with breath and focused energy.

Notes for the active partner: Try to give your sensation as quickly as possible. If pain is given in a flash, the receiver does not have a chance to tense up and the sensation is more pleasurable.

Notes for the receptive partner: Alternate calming and charging breaths. Make sounds. Move the energy with PC squeezes. Remember, you are in complete control of this experience. Go as far as you and your partner want to go, *and* observe your limits.

This is an experiment in how pain and intense sensation build erotic energy within you and between you and your partner. Try to release your expectations of what you think should happen as well as your desire to make something happen. Simply witness each present moment of the exercise.

As with the exercise in power, I strongly suggest you switch roles. Whether you are a top, a bottom, or a switch by nature, this experiment in how to move and transform pain into energy is a valuable (and delightful) exercise.

Now that you have a direct, mindful, solo and partnered experience of pain as an energetic force, feel free to add the sex. Sex is an especially delicious complement to pain. You can alternate deep thrusts and soft strokes with stinging blows. Spanking, nipple biting, and hair pulling make great accompaniments to fucking. Rake your fingernails over your lover's back, belly, and thighs. Pour the wax from a low-temperature paraffin candle on your beloved's back as you fuck them. Raid your kitchen for potential kinky toys. Keep a collection of wooden spoons, spatulas, fondue forks, and pickle tongs within easy reach. You can take one favorite sensation to new levels of intensity, or mix it up with varying intensities of sharp, pinchy, thuddy, stinging, hot and cold.

The endorphins and comfort provided by the sex provide the perfect lubricant for expanding levels of orgasmic pain. You can climb to ecstatic heights with pain, then slide down through the valleys with sex, then swoop back up on pain. Your only limits are your imagination and an eventual need for water, food, and sleep.

Now that you've visited the place on the erotic map where Tantric sex and BDSM intersect, don't be a stranger! Stop by often and explore all that the neighborhood has to offer. It's growing larger and more diverse every day.

Author's Note: The exercises in this chapter were adapted from workshop exercises I created in collaboration with Dossie Easton, coauthor of Radical Ecstasy: S/M Journeys Into Transcendence. *I am grateful to her for all I learned while cofacilitating these workshops and for all the fun I had learning it. I am also grateful to Kate Bornstein for her invaluable insights on the practice of solo pain.*

CHAPTER

8

PIERCING SCENES
FIFTHANGEL

When I am pierced, I feel like a little bit of my spirit is released from my body and is allowed to fly. The needle goes in, it's like a quick flash of pain, then a slow ache in my skin as it travels in, followed by another flash as the needle comes back out of my skin on the other side. I feel the light, the sensation, I open my eyes and I let go. Intimacy is shared, the outside world disappears, and we melt into each other, together.

—KATIE

Poking needles into flesh is one of my favorite things to do. Really. There are a variety of reasons why a person may want to perform temporary piercings on another. A top may pierce for the enjoyment of the bottom or for her reactions, which might not always be pleasant. Piercing is much more invasive than other types of SM skills. Whereas a flogging is an external kind of stimulation, with needles you are entering the body. This can feel like a different type of penetration to some or an invasion of the body to others, and piercing often creates a more intimate experience between partners. From an artistic viewpoint, piercing allows the top creative expression; one can create different designs with needle configurations and shapes, colors, decorative ribbon, and other items. Imagine putting feathers in the hubs of the needles after they have been placed and transforming your bottom into a peacock.

Some bottoms use piercing as an adjunct to a scene involving medical play, other temporary body modification, or blood play, while others may do it solely for the sensation of being pierced and its accompanying endorphin rush. Endorphins are morphine-like substances originating from within the body—the body's natural painkiller. Endorphins cause those feelings of exhilaration we get when we experience pain, stress, or excitement. When I pierce my own chest during a hook pull ritual, I get a sense of opening myself up on a deep level. Whether they are called chakras, loci, or meridians, different parts of the body hold special significance in certain spiritual beliefs and this can be accessed through piercing.

I took off my shirt and my bra and lay back on the bed. I was nervous, but he said he would walk me through it. I took a deep breath as he placed the first needle in my chest and exhaled as he pushed it through. I moaned in pleasure as the needle passed through my flesh. The adrenaline kicked in and I felt warm all over. My heart was racing. It made me feel beautiful. He kissed me deeply and caressed my body as I continued to moan and quiver. Sometimes physical pain is the best way to relieve emotional pain.

—MANDI

PIERCING SUPPLIES

Let's talk about the supplies you need to work with needles in a scene. Ideally, you need a bottom to poke, but you could start on yourself if you like. Besides needles and cleanup supplies, you'll need an understanding of basic anatomy and know how to prepare the skin, and you should know the medical history of the person you are piercing. Keep in mind that there are people out there who have needle phobias. They have an irrational fear of needles and will pass out in response to touching, being poked by, or even seeing needles. Trust me, it has happened in my classes.

When asking a partner about his or her medical history, find out if they have any allergies. Common allergies that pertain to needle work include allergies to latex and to iodine or shellfish. If the bottom has an allergy to latex, you will want to use nitrile or vinyl gloves. Should you encounter a shellfish/iodine allergy, use a skin prep other than Povidone-iodine. Also inquire about bleeding disorders and the use of blood-thinning medications. These do not necessarily disqualify a person from having needles put into them, but you should take into consideration bruising and make sure any bleeding has stopped.

Skin Prep

In order to prepare the skin and decrease the risk of infection when using needles, you should use a skin prep solution. There are many types—some are more readily available, and some may be more cost effective. I personally like to use Chlorhexidine. However, any of the preparations discussed below will work; just be sure to follow the manufacturer's directions for use as skin prep. Some of these come as a solution that you can apply with sterile gauze pads; some are also available as individually wrapped pads with the solution on them.

- **61% ethyl alcohol**
  Ethyl alcohol is commonly found in antibacterial hand soap; you can buy 61% solution at your local pharmacy.

- **Povidone-iodine**
  The most common brand name of this solution is Betadine, and it can be found in drugstores. If the bottom is allergic to shellfish or iodine, *do not use* Povidone-iodine. Note: this solution will temporarily discolor the skin.

- **70% isopropyl alcohol**
  This is the least expensive solution on the list and the easiest to find in drugstores; however, in medical studies, it's also the least effective at killing bacteria found on the skin.

- **6% benzocaine with isopropyl alcohol 70%**
  The same as above, but this product also numbs the skin a little.

- **Chlorhexidine**
  Chlorhexidine comes in 2% or 4% concentrations or a 1% concentration combined with 61% ethyl alcohol. You can purchase these at your local pharmacy or from online medical suppliers.

Gloves

There are many types of gloves out there, but I tend to use nitrile gloves because they are latex free and I can get them in purple. Purple is the color of the hanky for piercing, should you wish to do any flagging. I find latex gloves more stretchy and easier to put on. Nitrile and vinyl gloves, though latex free, are harder to put on, especially if your hands get moist from sweating or if you are changing gloves frequently. You may find that some bottoms react poorly to the sight of blood. Black gloves are available, often used by tattoo artists and piercing shops, that decrease the visibility of blood on the gloves, should things get a little messy. For you folks who are all into the "black look," these would enhance your wardrobe.

Cleanup Supplies

When you are using needles, you may encounter blood, so always have cleanup supplies handy. Don't make things too complicated. You can use plain paper towels to clean up the holes. If inclined to do so, you can treat each hole as a trauma wound and tape gauze pads to each one. To clean work surfaces, use a 10% household bleach solution and paper towels. Make this solution by mixing one and a half cups of household bleach and a gallon of water, or one part bleach to nine parts water. Make sure you are wearing gloves when working with bleach. Bleach begins to lose its effectiveness in a short period of time, so discard the bleach after your cleanup. Make a new batch of bleach solution if you do not use it within 24 hours.

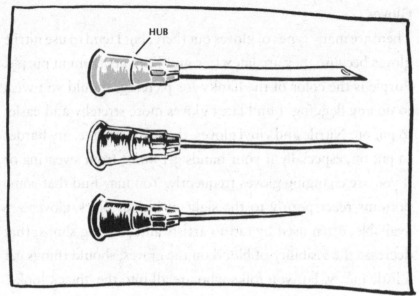

Illustration 8.1. Piercing needles

Needles

Needles come in a plethora of sizes (or gauges), the most common being 25, 23, 22, 20, and 18. They are measured by their diameter: the larger the number, the smaller the diameter. Thus an 18-gauge needle is a larger-diameter needle (1.270 mm outside diameter) than a 25-gauge (0.508 mm outside diameter). Additionally, needles come in varying lengths, the most common being ⅝ inch, 1 inch, and 1½ inch. Use only single-use disposable needles in sterile packaging.

For the most part, you will want to use "hubbed" needles, as they are the most commonly available, cheapest to buy, and have the bonus feature of a "handle" which aids placement of the needle (See Illustration 8.1: Piercing needles.) Another name for this type of needle is *hypodermic*, from Greek, meaning under the skin. Hub needles can be obtained from online medical supply stores or fetish supply stores. Be sure you are abiding by your local laws concerning the purchase of needles. Other needle types include acupuncture, spinal, TB, insulin, body piercing, Huber, and biopsy.

HOW TO PIERCE

When I am pierced, I have the sensation that I'm flying—I feel simultaneously grounded and floaty. I love the very intimate invasion of personal space that piercing produces, the involuntary giggling, the contact high. I love the air of danger, of doing something that others deem "too out there," and loving it. I love to see fresh red blood, not the least bit oxidized yet, trailing down my flesh and the patterns it makes as it soaks into a sheet.

—AMY

Beginning piercers should stick to fleshy places like the chest, back, arms, and legs. Basically, if you can pinch the skin and not feel muscle between your fingers, it is okay to put a needle there. Until you are more experienced and have gained more education, avoid piercing the genitals, face, neck, tongue or other less fleshy areas of the body. Some bottoms may feel more at ease if they are able to watch; others are horrified to watch. Pick what is right for the scene.

When you are prepping the skin, use the recommendations provided by the manufacturer of the product you are using.

Pinch a section of skin between your fingers. Insert the needle parallel to the surface of the skin. (See Illustration 8.2: Needle insertion.) Using this technique, you prevent the needle from penetrating anything vital. How close you pierce to the body determines how much of the needle will be in the skin and how deep the needle will be buried. Also, you must take into account the length of your needle. If you want the tip of the needle to come back out of the skin, you need to pierce higher up on your pinch and farther away from the body.

Grasp the needle with your dominant hand, using your thumb and index finger to hold the needle by its hub. Line up the needle parallel to the surface of the skin next to the place you have pinched, and be sure that your fingertips are far enough away that you are not going to poke yourself when the needle comes out the other side. Bottoms may jump in response to the initial poke or squirm as you push the needle through the skin. Anticipate this movement to avoid poking yourself. Some piercers leave the pointy end of the needle inside the skin after they have placed it. This can keep you from getting poked by a "dirty" needle (one that has already been used) if you are placing needles close together.

Some piercers put needles through fast, while others push slowly. The choice is yours—each way produces a different sensation. Larger-gauge needles, 12 and above, may require a sterile lubricant to aid their insertion.

You will soon discover that not everyone's skin is the same. Some people have thin skin, which makes piercing very easy, while others have thick, tough skin requiring a sledgehammer to drive the needle in. The thicker the skin, the more difficult it is to pinch. Coating the needle with sterile lube may help you with needle placement in tough skin.

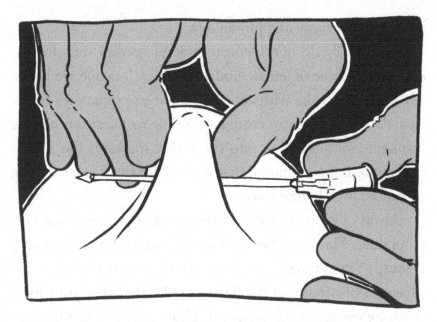

Illustration 8.2. Needle insertion

OTHER CONSIDERATIONS

One factor to consider is room temperature. A warmer room is more conducive to people passing out in response to needles, so you may want to think about that if you have a bottom with a fear of needles. Heating up the room to keep your bottom warm might be a bad idea. Besides, a cold room can make the nipples erect and easier to pierce—when you get more pokes under your belt. (Okay, I might have a nipple fetish.)

If you poke needles straight down into the skin—that is, perpendicular to the skin surface, you run the risk of poking organs such as the lungs, heart, intestines, liver, and spleen. This is especially true with longer needles. Stick to the simple technique of pinching the skin unless you have studied human anatomy. If you want to be a great piercer, take a college course in anatomy and physiology.

I especially do not advocate poking needles straight into the breast tissue of female-bodied people. (Imagine the breast as a birthday cake with candles). There are structures in the female breast that are more susceptible to infection; placing puncture wounds deep into the breast increases the risk of infection. It is my opinion that women who are breast-feeding are at an even higher risk.

Always dispose of your needles in a puncture-proof plastic container. Many people just use commercially manufactured "sharps" containers, but some local ordinances allow for disposal of needles in regular trash. Please check your local laws concerning needle disposal. Many public dungeons often have specific containers for disposal of bloody materials such as paper towels and gloves.

HOW THE BODY REACTS TO PIERCING

Bottoms can react in different ways to piercing. Those who enjoy piercing will welcome the sensation and be receptive to it. Some may get very still, while others may thrash about. It is best to talk to your bottom and discuss how he may react. Remember that piercing is unlike some other SM activities in that a fear of needles is a common phobia. Let's face it: most of our first experiences with needles were in a medical office—not the best introduction to piercing and needles. With a person who has never been pierced before, always prepare for the worst, but be open to everything. You cannot always predict how someone's body will react to needles.

One evening my wife, Katie, and I were having sex in our home dungeon. Katie and I had been together for about four years at the time and I had yet to place needles in her nipples. This seemed like a great time to address that oversight. By this point Katie was really hating me—at anything I did she screamed "No!" and fought back in anger. I should add that Katie and I are very experienced at what we do. She often protests during our scenes—it's part of how we do BDSM. As I inserted a single needle into each nipple, you would have thought I was cutting a limb off. If she had not been rendered immobile, I think she would have run out of the house naked.

So what size needles did I put in her nipples? It may surprise you to know that I used 25-gauge ⅝-inch needles. Keep in mind that Katie has no problems with needles in general—I have poked her hundreds of times, but her nipples are borderline hypersensitive. When I proposed marriage to her, she was suspended from six 8-gauge hooks in her back. So why did she have such a violent reaction to these tiny, tiny things in her nipples? The answer is context, location, and pain theory. When it comes to needle work, size really does not matter, nor does the number of needles you place.

There is a theory called "wind-up" that pertains to pain and the body's response to pain. Wind-up pain results from the constant bombardment of the neurons in the spinal cord. Pain becomes amplified and the body develops opioid tolerance: opioid painkillers are no longer effective. If pain goes untreated during surgery, for example, wind-up can occur, causing the patient to wake up with increased sensitivity to pain. Additionally, the body's own natural responses to pain no longer work.

All that adrenaline and those endorphins go right out the door. This may be an "aha" moment for some of you.

Taking this into account, I knew that I did not have to place harpoons into Katie's nipples to get the sexual satisfaction I wanted. This understanding about the body's response to pain enabled me to avoid the potential complications of greater trauma or damage caused by larger-gauge needles in such a small target. Yeah, I did fuck her one more time after the needles were in place, but I held her for a long time after it was over—she was in a rather fragile emotional state.

THE RISKS

When you puncture someone's skin, you must be aware of the potential dangers. If you slide a needle into someone, then accidentally poke yourself as it comes out the other side, you can be exposed to their blood. The most common potentially infectious body fluids are: blood, preseminal fluid (precum), semen, vaginal secretions, and any fluid in which blood can be seen (for example, bloody saliva after brushing teeth). Exposure can be defined as an incident when the potentially infectious blood or body fluids of one person come in contact with the blood or body fluids of another. If these fluids come into contact with cuts or sores, hangnails, needle sticks, or mucous membranes, there is the potential for exposure. Mucous membranes are those linings or cavities of the human body that are exposed to air: the linings of the digestive tract and the mouth, respiratory tract and nose, conjunctiva of the eyes, and the genitourinary tract, including the urethra. Contact of potentially infectious body fluids with intact skin does not constitute exposure.

The bloodborne pathogens that are of greatest concern are the hepatitis B and C viruses (HBV and HCV) and Human Immunodeficiency Virus (HIV). Blood contains the highest concentrations of HBV, HCV, and HIV, thus contact with blood poses the highest risk of transmission.

Based on 2005 statistics, the known risk for becoming infected with HIV after a percutaneous exposure (needle stick) to blood containing HIV is approximately 0.3 percent—that is, 1 out of 300 exposures will result in seroconversion. The rate for hepatitis B-positive seroconversion in a nonimmunized host is 6 to 24 percent and for exposure to hepatitis C, 1 to 10 percent.

Hepatitis B and C

When contracted, hepatitis attacks the liver and can result in lifelong illness. Liver cancer, failure of the liver, permanent scarring of the liver called cirrhosis, and death can occur after a person has become infected with HBV or HCV.

A carrier is an individual who is infected by the virus and has not recovered fully from infection. They may harbor the virus for the rest of their life without any signs or symptoms of infection. The only way to know if you are infected with HBV or HCV is to get a blood test.

A virus needs a host such as a human to live in. Many viruses do not survive long outside the human body. HCV can stay alive in a drop of blood for up to four days. HBV is a rather strong "bug" that can live in a drop of blood for about a week. Hepatitis B and C are easier to acquire than HIV for this reason.

There is an HBV vaccine available. It consists of a series of three injections given over a six-month period. I recommend that all persons involved in BDSM activities get the series.

HIV/AIDS

HIV is the virus that causes Acquired Immune Deficiency Syndrome (AIDS). It is a rather weak virus compared to HBV, in that it is easily destroyed outside the human body. HIV is less contagious than HBV or HCV because there are lower concentrations of HIV in a drop of blood. However, there is still a serious risk of transmission. The stage of infection affects the concentrations of the virus in body fluids—the more advanced the illness, the higher the concentration of the virus. Currently there is no approved HIV vaccine.

What to Do if You Have Been Exposed

Should an exposure occur, remain calm. If you stick yourself with a needle that has been used on another person, or are otherwise exposed, immediate treatment is essential.

For exposure as a result of broken skin, clean the exposed area with soap and water. Squeezing blood out of the wound has no added effect.

If exposure is to the mucous membranes, flush the affected area with water for 15 minutes.

Contact your primary care physician immediately. If there has been possible exposure to HBV, medical treatment needs to begin within 24 hours. Opinions vary as to when prophylaxis treatment should begin for possible exposure to HIV: from 30 minutes to 4 hours has been recommended.

Exposure to infectious diseases must be taken very seriously—they can be life-threatening. Get tested for HBV, HCV, and HIV for your own sake and for the safety of those you scene with. Positive HBV, HCV, or HIV status does not preclude future scenes involving blood so long as standard precautions are taken. Be open to your partners concerning your medical status. It is inexcusable to have an infectious disease and not tell your partner about it.

NEEDLE WORK AFTERCARE

If a wound is going to become infected, it will usually happen in the first 24 to 72 hours. This statistic is based on infections arising from open-wound trauma that required closure. Infection rates for a "clean wound," such as the ones created from operating on intact skin without entering any internal organs, is 2.5 percent. These rates are compiled from surgical incisions, not tiny holes from a needle. What you are doing is puncturing normal healthy tissue. To prevent infection, clean the area twice a day with clean gauze and a mixture of equal parts hydrogen peroxide and water. (It's not necessary to use sterile gauze.) If desired, and if there is no allergy, apply Neosporin to the area one to three times a day.

Consult a physician if you develop any of these signs and symptoms of infection:

- Slight redness around the insertion site is normal, but redness should not spread beyond the site. Red streaking leading away from the wound is a definite sign of infection.

- Pain and tenderness and mild bruising are normal, but the pain and swelling should be greatest during the second day and should then diminish.
- Increased redness or warmth
- Any drainage from the site
- Any fever above 100.4 degrees Fahrenheit

PIERCING IN A SCENE

I love everything about play piercing: the desire to develop and maintain an advanced skill, the intense intimacy during the scene, the visceral animalistic emotions brought on by blood, and the satisfaction of pleasing my partner. Piercing play requires trust between partners, and the feelings of vulnerability, anticipation, and the power exchange provide just as much of a rush for the piercer as the physical sensations do for the one being pierced. There is an element of performance art to it as well. I do not consider myself an artist, but when working with needles and a willing exhibitionist, I can explore that part of my personality.

—DOUG

Please keep in mind that this is an introduction to needle work. There are many places to go from here. You can combine needles with other types of scenes—here are just a few ideas. To add some more pain to the equation, spray 70% isopropyl alcohol on the fresh piercing holes to make them sting. If your bottom likes humiliation, have him walk around a public dungeon all bandaged up or with a hundred elastic bandages stuck all over his body. Piercing can easily be combined with virtually any other type of scene. Once a person is in bondage, needles can be placed anywhere that you can access skin. The needles themselves can be used for bondage by looping a string around the ends and attaching the other end of the string to a stationary object.

For a more artistic flair, needles can be placed to create various shapes and designs. Some folks layer the needles to make a "button." This is accomplished by inserting a needle in regular fashion and then inserting another needle just under the first, but at a 90-degree angle to it—think of a pinwheel. Multiple needles can be placed in the same area using this technique. Just use one of the needles you already inserted to lift up the skin to ease placement of subsequent needles. After the needles are in place you can press on the "button" with a gloved hand or finger to increase the intensity of the piercing. Be extra careful not to get poked. After you've pierced the flesh and the sharp end of the needle has come out the other side, you can carefully put the end into a sterile cork or decorative "cap"—it's a great way to prevent getting poked.

Are you getting the idea that there is more to needle work than simply placing the needles? Of course there are more things to do to up the excitement. Rotating the needles, pulling on the needles, and using larger-gauge needles are ways to be a little more sadistic. Just use your imagination and have fun.

I want to share one more thing about the story I told earlier. As I write this, Katie and I are waiting for her nipple jewelry to arrive. You see, Katie asked me to permanently pierce her nipples. But she gets to watch me do it. Funny how that worked out.

CHAPTER 9

BRUTAL AFFECTION: PLAYING WITH ROUGH SEX

FELICE SHAYS

The sweet intersection of slap and kiss. The rough and tumble of pound and caress, of commanding voice and gentle stroke, of laugh and growl. Welcome to the intense and gorgeous world of rough sex.

Rough sex is not one person deciding desires and limits. Rough sex is not one person accepting whatever is done to them or when it stops. Rough sex is not polite. Rough sex is not abuse. Rough sex is not payback or punishment.

Rough sex is consent and desire.

Rough sex treads on taboos, giving them a wink and the finger.

Rough sex is the clear permission to take and give power.

Rough sex doesn't care about what gender you are, how

you look, who you fuck, or who others say you're supposed to be.

Rough sex is release, dominance, resistance, objectification, humiliation, imagination, role play, giving in, giving over.

Rough sex is connected, laughing, loving, silly, growling, playful.

Rough sex is awareness, calculating, tender, self-confident, respectful.

Rough sex is primal, raw, spiritual, animalistic, unruly, breathless, ruthless, famished, predatory, ecstatic.

Rough sex is unfolding and claiming your desire.

Rough sex is using your hands, genitals, mouth, heart, toys, and brain.

Rough sex is passion and ache.

In this chapter, we will explore how to find and express your own desire, push through fears, communicate, negotiate, and define your physical and emotional limits and release. Plus, I'll let you in on a compelling assortment of techniques, ideas, and safety tips so you can get busy expressing *your* brutal affection.

CLAIMING YOUR DESIRES

There are lots of reasons why people want to have fierce, power-imbued, consensual sex. Say you lead a complicated life that requires you to make endless decisions and keep control of your home, work, or school. The opportunity for someone who respects you, likes you, or loves you to come in and "relieve you" of your power by running the show for a few hours is liberating. Maybe you've always been a scrappy kid—wrestling with your sisters and brothers and the kids at school. To feel the force from someone aching to be pounded into by you, or they into you, feels like being put back into your flesh in a most exquisite way. Perhaps, for you, gentle is only part of your story. Expressing physically the power, passion, and heat you carry is what links you to your lover and connects you both in a spiritual, emotional way that tenderness doesn't always reach. Maybe it's more primal: you like to slap people while fucking them with all your strength. You get rock hard and slippery wet fantasizing about being tied spread-eagled to the kitchen table, gagged and blindfolded. Like other kinds of BDSM, rough sex releases endorphins—chemicals from the brain which block pain and create feelings of euphoria; many people thrill at the rush and high they feel from intense physical sensations.

Something shifts in me. Something shuts off—some internal voice is silenced. I don't see my stretch marks, or the dirty clothes on the floor. No, I'm aware of something shoving the critics out of the way, displacing them. To think this is only about body parts is a mistake. It's like my brain gets quieted by the roar of my hunger, ache, need. I take what I want knowing she wants me to take her again and again. I become so tall and strong—like a mother pushing a car off a baby stuck in a stroller. It is absolutely a spiritual undertaking. Not like god but yes, like god. Tapping into an essence that only comes when you let go—when you are relieved of your life in its everyday trappings and wrappings.

Mainstream society delivers a constant barrage of restrictive, prescriptive, and often conflicting messages. Although ads and movies are filled with images of rough sex, it is still considered deviant behavior. We're taught confusing lessons like Have, desire, and love one partner forever; Make yourself sexy to your man but don't be a slut; Desire what everyone else does; Strike out and be an individual—but don't deviate too far from what is acceptable.

None of these precepts translate well to the bedroom or to creating an arsenal of fantasies. Even the powerful, long sought after achievements of feminist equality that must be intrinsic in a society committed to equality can sometimes wreak havoc in our sex lives. When you first get together with someone, the unknown newness of the other creates an erotic tension that is the cornerstone of sexual desire. Over time the ease, equality, and comfort we strive for in our intimate relationships can be the very undoing to this necessary positive tension. Add roughing up or being roughed up by this person you love and with whom you derive comfort, and it's easy to feel confused.

Rough sex demands respect and equal voice—even if that's not how it looks when you're in it. Fantasizing or craving to be "raped" by your lover does not make you a sick person. You don't need to be cured of anything. You might need therapy for other reasons, but getting off on someone calling you "a filthy set of holes" doesn't necessarily signify deep, unresolved psychological issues. On the other hand, *being belittled or denied the things you need and want at the hands of your lover is not foreplay—it's abuse. Being violent with someone who has said no in any form is abuse. Actual rape is an invasion and a crime.*

"How Do I Figure Out What I Want?"

The biggest challenge in the search to discover and name your desire is keeping an open mind. Do not judge yourself or think that what you want is perverted or wrong; silence the voice in your head that tells you you're alone in your desire, or that your lover (or potential lover) will reject you. Don't apologize for your desire. And don't confuse fantasy with reality. As long as your fantasy of seducing the newspaper boy is acted out with another consenting adult, you're lucky to be in touch with your desire. And no, you're not messed up.

For the past decade I've taught and worked with thousands of people across North America who occupy radically different places in the world: in their experiences, in their proclivities and repulsions, in how they look, who they like to be sexual with, and how they get off. (Long ago, when I learned that one of my then new kinky friends worked as a flight attendant, my world shifted on its axis. Now every time I fly I assume there is a raucous lover serving me my peanuts.) But regardless of class, level of education, gender, and orientation, one question always comes up: How do I figure out what I want?

Start with what you already know you like: being pinned down while being fucked, say, or squeezing your balls to the point of pain when you come. Let your mind wander. In a fantasy, what might come before and after that? Do not edit or censor yourself. Write it down.

Go to your local sex toy store in person or online and peruse book and DVD titles that you find intriguing. Remember, there is an inexhaustible flow of bravado and misrepresentation online and in porn. Get ideas, be turned on or horrified—just don't think you are supposed to be that bendable, invincible, or stretch that wide! Check out the resource guide at the back of this book to find a plethora of smart, reliable websites and educators filled with intelligent, responsible, sexy ideas and information.

Do any of your friends talk about or allude to being into rough stuff (whatever that means to them)? There are far more "naughty" people out there than you might imagine. When you find chat rooms and like-minded people, don't only lurk—engage, ask questions, answer queries, challenge, listen. If you are trying to suss this out in tandem with your partner, the process is similar: each of you discovering and revealing what makes you squirm is half the fun. Share links and images (I'm a fan of "I want this" images sent via text or email, or left in the medicine cabinet). Read erotica to each other, or using different-colored ink, take turns underlining passages in a shared book. This idea works because you don't have to say out loud what might feel too embarrassing at first. Ask your partner to write a list of turn-ons—from the benign to the hard-core. You can compare notes or just certain parts if revealing the whole list might be too scary.

COMMUNICATION AND NEGOTIATION

I love when you, my lover, let me be small—yes, let me— because I know you will respect me and my limits, hold me, without judgment, keep me safe. We think each other the hottest things on two feet (we tell each other so often—and not just in bed). So even when, during sex, you are calling me names, or fucking me so hard, or pushing me to take more, you know it's exactly what I crave. Thank God we've talked about this so often. I love your ferocity and won't let you hurt me in ways I don't want to be hurt. Please, take care of everything for a while; know where we are driving. Yes, I will help pay for gas, help you decide the route, but you drive and I will let go.

I'm hungry to keep you safe and hold you strong. Push you to see that you are mighty and tender and can take yourself even further than you ever thought you could. I have told you countless times how I adore you and think you are breathlessly sexy, and you too tell me that I'm crazy hot so we don't need to do that now. During sex I may call you names or hold you down; we've talked about all of this already. I know it makes you weak with need—hell, me too. I can give you sensations that rough up your brain and release endorphins. And you can know that I'm driving. Trust that I know where we are going or at least when we need a rest stop. And though I'm holding the wheel, I don't for a minute stop glorying at the scenery. And you—you can let go.

It doesn't matter if you are hooking up for a night or a lifetime, *the one non-negotiable element is permission*—getting it and respecting it.

If you're on the receiving end of rough play, remember that you are not a passive vessel. If you want something harder, faster, slower, started or stopped—tell your lover. "Oh god, yes!" counts as feedback. So does "Ow, stop, wait. Damn, that's big. Let's try this, baby." You are not timid or imperfect for speaking up. On the contrary, you are proving yourself to be a trusted lover who is committed to having connected, hot sex. Nothing changes unless you make it change. And though it looks as if the person who is meting out the roughness is in power, that is just the opposite of what's happening. The one being roughed up is the one who has the final word about what does and doesn't happen.

If you're doling out the rough play, you are not a fucking machine, aiming to please only yourself or your lover. Start slowly, building up and discovering your own and your partner's desire and tolerance for more intensity. If you go from zero to 60 in no time flat, your lover may not be able to keep up, or be interested in it. Someone giving herself to you is a gift; take your time discovering what's inside. This does not mean that a slow buildup is an "always" rule. Sometimes, you need to throw someone against a wall and take what you want. Pinning his hands to his side, you clamp down on his neck with your mouth and bite—long and hard. Sometimes, while his cock is in you, you reach your arms up and pound his back with your fist as he growls and leans down to kiss you. But you know jumping into it at full speed is right for both of you because together you have experimented, talked, and listened with clarity and respect.

"Now That I Know, How Do I Get What I Want?"
All relationships, whether you've been together 10 minutes or 10 years, have radically different histories of experience, trust, and disappointment, but the basics of getting clear, brave, and open are the same. Do you know what it is you want? Have you articulated specific activities to yourself? Have you experienced things with a previous lover that you want with this partner? It's okay to have only a sense of what you want—just remember that your partner can't know till you know. Getting what you want in any avenue of life involves risk. You and your sex are worth it. Over a drink, on a walk, or on the subway, say a thing or two that you love about your sex or sensuality together. Say something you want to try. You can also (but you don't have to) have a lengthy talk or write a list of what you want or don't want.

Talking can be sexy—sometimes simply introducing the idea unlocks the taboo door. "I love it when I'm going down on you and you hold my head exactly where you want it—not letting me move around a lot." Or "Remember that scene in the movie where he pushed her against the car, slapped her face, and then kissed her? Oh my God, that was hot." Bring home erotica or porn with stories or images that turn you on. Share it with your lover on a date. Ask what she thinks about when she masturbates. Tell her what you think about too.

Talk a little, fuck a lot, talk some more. Be ready to use your words during your sex—this is where the other part of the conversation can happen. You pin him down, sitting on his belly, and bite his nipple slow and hard. Pause, ask, "Is this okay? You like it? You feel so good under me."

It's important to realize, however, that new lovers can't rely solely on during-sex talk—ego and fear of rejection or disapproval easily skew communication. Even if you've been together a long time, you're still (or sometimes more) susceptible to the challenges of being clear and accurate about needs and wants during sex. Longtime lovers' dynamics may be so engrained that in-bed talk proves to be insufficient. Maybe you've been together a while and you want your sex to be less predictable and more primal. She's a great lover, but you feel that something's missing. Maybe it's a general attitude shift you ache for. Lots of people want their partners to be more domineering—run the show, make decisions, be more aggressive. Other folks want to turn the tables on what have become established roles. How lovers discuss potentially thorny topics (politics, finances, family, etc.) is generally how they will approach talking about sex; the more skilled the communicators, the better the sex.

The more you know what you want, the easier it is to put it out there. However, if you have a narrow set of ideas that *must* happen or a specific script that *must* be followed, you cut your partner out of the decision-making process. Stay open to ideas and changes. Start by talking about what turns you on about your partner's body, her sex responses, and your sex together. Yes, talking so specifically about sex can feel risky and vulnerable. This becomes further compounded when you articulate your desire for taboo or aggressive sex; it's intellectually and emotionally confusing to crave this with the same person you hold to be solid and safe.

Watch. Listen. Talk.

"Let's get real—talking does *not* equal spontaneity."

Are you someone who believes that rough sex means just going for it? I get it. Going for it is *hot*. Theoretically. Suppose you serve a beautiful candlelit dinner complete with soufflé to your date only to discover she's allergic to eggs. You worked hard but you both end up feeling kinda crappy—and hungry. The ambience is still wonderful, but had you (even briefly) talked about what food you eat and love, the feasting might have lasted long into the night. Or you meet at a party, you talk, you flirt, you lean in and say, "I want to slam into you, bring you to your knees, and make you forget there's a god" and your prey looks at you, smiling, and holds out his hand to you. (a) You're a lucky dog. (b) You two just communicated a common desire. You talked. And it's still spontaneous.

Without any kind of preliminary talk, if you just "go for it" you might get your rocks off, but will you please your lover? Will you hurt your lover? How will you know? If both of you don't care (though determining this is difficult at best), more power to you—really, I support this fully. Hopefully there won't be any physical or emotional fallout later.

Most people, however, do care how each other feels. But if you ask your date *during* your passionate sex if he wants and likes what's going on, you might not get a truthful answer, out of shyness or reluctance to offend. With new lovers especially, once the action gets hot, fair and equal negotiation is harder to come by, especially on the first or second date. (Hell, it's hard enough with long-term lovers.) Each of you is trying to impress and suss out the other, bringing your best game and sexiest moves; nerves mar perception. The power imbalance exists—and it's tipped toward the one who's doing the roughing up. Even willing participants have tough times speaking up if something is going awry; no one wants to be seen as a prude or a wimp. A little talk before you get busy can change all that.

And you know what? Right now you can commit to speaking honestly and simply and not accusatorily about what you want and don't want. Owning your stuff—figuring out how to communicate—frees us in every aspect of our lives. Do it—you don't have to live anything but a shiny, bold life.

ROLES, CHANGE, AND CONFIDENCE

Let's say you want to be submissive but your partner isn't confident or comfortable in a dominating role. What to do? Is your partner into the idea but doesn't know where to start? Have you brought it up in the past and it's fallen flat? You might have a good idea of what your submissive role looks and sounds like—maybe you've fantasized about it often enough that you have a specific sexy script or two. This is perfect for masturbation but not always successful for coupling up. Tell your partner you want to explore her being more dominating. *Some* specifics are needed and then the parlay begins.

Experimentation works far better than expectations. She doesn't need to run out and buy a big flogger or have you kneeling tonight and calling her Mistress (though she might). Instead, the two of you come up with a list of what the action might look like, including your fantasies. Start simple—she sits on top of you and pins your arms to your sides with her knees, not letting you touch her or her cunt. Keep it playful. Though there is no guarantee your partner will ever be as dominant as you fantasize or will wield sexual power over you in the ways your fantasies map out, there is no guarantee that she won't either. Stay open—surprise each other.

Perhaps your partner has asked you to take on a role you don't usually take. First, ask yourself, do you *want* to take on the role? Or is this solely your partner's desire? If indeed you want to try a new role or position, keep your mind open as to what it might be. Is it a generic positioning (I want you to dominate me) or is it a specific role (you're the school principal and I'm the troublemaker student). If your partner, say, wants you to initiate and dominate when you have mostly been the receiver or equal, talk with her—get details and examples. The fact that you're already talking about it means you're off to a good, sexy start. The fantasy in your partner's head can help, but it can also hinder if she is too attached to the specifics and trying to fit you to them. If parts of the description resonate with you, start with one or two actions and weave them into your sex. If a role feels too cookie-cutter or stereotyped and doesn't ring true for you, neither of you may get much pleasure from it.

Take five minutes on your own and (yep, corny) write down everything you think of when you imagine that role. Don't edit. You might find laughter or goofiness on that list. Leave a sex toy, panties, or other piece of clothing with instructions for your lover. Email, text, IM, snail mail, write notes, or Skype your provocative invitations. Whatever resonates in you is where you begin your exploration of any new role. Let it grow and morph from there. If and when you get stuck, write as often as it's useful. And whatever else you uncover, remember that desire and consent are the cornerstones of all rough sex.

ACTIVITIES, IDEAS, AND TECHNIQUES

You've talked, you've fantasized, you've plotted and conspired. Now what? Some activities that meet under the large umbrella that is rough sex include: face slapping, biting, hitting, pushing, pounding penetration, denying touch or orgasm, spitting, punching, spanking, gagging, name calling, and bondage. Folks also like to control-kiss, choke, and push or shove a bottom down on the bed, slam a bottom against a wall, pinch nipples, balls, and labia, grab and squeeze thighs/ass/upper arms/wrists, pull hair, force a bottom's face into a pillow, control breathing, talk smut, rip off clothing, and claim "ownership" of someone. Here are some delicious tips, ideas, techniques, and safety precautions you can incorporate into your rough sex play.

Restraining Your Lover

> *It's a huge turn-on when a guy is pinning you down and you can just tell how bad he wants you. When it gets to that point where it feels like if you don't get that person you're seriously going to die on that bed, it's hot. It's needing someone in a really different way. And it's insanely hot when you can see a guy feeling that way. Even if it's only sex—not love or commitment or anything like that. It's all about that moment. And the only thing he wants is you and he is seriously rabid to have you.*
>
> —Chasing the Jersey[1]

Tied spread-eagled to a headboard. Hands holding down arms. Pinned against a crumbling alley wall. Struggling to get free. Bondage and restraints. Our fantasies and sex are filled with all that and more. Luckily, this book has a chapter by Midori on how to do bondage and do it well. Let's just touch on a just a few elements of restraint.

For all the reasons why rough sex is so prevalent and hot, the taboo desire to be held captive, without control or knowledge of what might happen to you, engages us just as fiercely. To deny someone (or to be denied of) something you really want, when you know you will get it sooner or later, can be sweet torture. Especially when the prize is sex.

Scarves, ties, rope, chain, leather belts, stockings, bedsheets—the materials that can be used to bind a lover are as endless as your imagination. Some are better than others, however. Silk scarves, though sensuous, knot quickly, easily, but are hell to unknot. Cheap handcuffs close further than they should and often get stuck. (Plus, "Oh my God! Where's the key?" is the last thing you want to hear.) Both of these kinds of restraints can dig into wrists and ankles and cut off circulation; they should be avoided. If you do use scarves or other fabric to bind wrists or ankles, have medical or bandage scissors ready—they have a flat side intended to slide between the bind and the skin without hurting while cutting the bind. If you use handcuffs, pin the key(s) on a nearby bulletin board, curtain, or door frame; don't leave them on the bedside table.

No matter what you tie your lover to—a bed, table, steering wheel, or tent stakes—make sure you've got the means to release your willing prey easily and quickly. This is also a great time for both of you to be ready to use a safeword or gesture in case of fear, pain, or emergency.

But you don't need "stuff" to keep someone where you want him. The craving to be physically controlled can be managed by placing your knees, hands, feet, and body onto your lover in strategic positions. Avoid joint-to-joint pressure (for instance, your knees on his wrists); aim rather for the more muscular and meatier parts of the body, such as forearms and thighs. Using your legs, knees, and feet to press on him frees up your hands to slap, punch, fuck, stroke, or get busy with a dildo and harness. And don't limit yourself to the bedroom: there are perfectly good walls, floors, picnic tables, trees, bathroom stalls, and movie seats aching for your play.

And finally, one of the most powerful methods of restraint doesn't use any physical means at all. It's your voice. "Keep that pretty mouth open." "I don't want to see you looking at me." "Good boy, you're sitting exactly where I left you." When both people are into it, this is intoxicating.

Hair Pulling

Weave your hand into a fist in the hair underneath the back of the head. Hold and pull by the roots. Grabbing any other part of the hair can cause the hair to rip from the scalp, causing distracting, undesired pain. You can lead your lover where you want her by this technique. If the receiver is on top, this is a great way to tip your willing prey back to fuck deeply. Use caution; don't jerk the neck or head.

Spitting

In some cultures, spitting is seen as the deepest of insults. Regardless of where you live, spitting saliva on or at someone is disgusting at worst or humiliating at best. Yes, I said at best. There are lots of people whose kink has them hungry to be objectified, humiliated, and degraded *in a sexy context*. Desiring this is not a mark of low self-esteem as long as the parties involved don't let this dynamic leak into nonsex situations. Spitting on or getting spit in the face, on the chest or breasts, or in the mouth are the definition of sexy to more people than you might imagine. Sometimes simply *because* it is considered so unacceptable, the shock of this unpredictable act can cement a sought-after power dynamic into place.

Some folks use saliva as lube—forget it. It dries up quickly and does nothing for the receiver. It might work to ease some friction for a hand job on a penis or dildo, but that's about where its usefulness ends. Saliva itself is not known to carry HIV. It is possible, however, to transmit STIs if there is blood in the saliva due to cuts or sores in the mouth.

As with every other sex activity in this book, don't knock it if you've never tried it. You never know…

Rough Blow Jobs

Blow jobs on a cock or dildo can be filthy hot and can be used in rough sex in endless ways. For example:

- Steer his head by his hair as he sucks your dick. Lift his mouth off you to spit on his face, kiss his pretty mouth, slap his face, tell him how good a job he's doing, what a worthless whore he is and not worth the money you've given him. Let him breathe as you gently stroke his face. Rinse and repeat.

- Pin her head against the wall or floor, or tell her to lie on her back, her head draped over the side of the bed. Fuck her face. Make her masturbate at the same time.

- Bind him to a chair by his hands and feet, legs spread wide. Suck his cock, bringing him almost to climax but not quite. Let him squirm against the butt plug.

- Put a butt plug in your ass and another one in his and because you both love to share, suck each other off simultaneously.

Deep Throat

Sometimes considered the holy grail by both the giver (the sucker) and receiver (the suckee), taking someone's cock fully in your mouth down to the balls is definitely hot, both physically and visually. It's also not always physiologically possible. The length, shape, and thickness of the cock or dildo and how wide the jaw can open are important considerations. To avoid gagging, drop the back of your palate as if your throat was yawning. Can't or don't want to take that big thing in your mouth? Wrap one hand around the base of the shaft and push your mouth down only far enough to meet your hand. This is a great visual, it jerks him off at the same time, and the giver only takes what she can in her throat. Winners, all.

Some people like to gag; they really get off on the gagging sounds, seeing the tears from the giver's eyes as the air is choked out of him, and the long threads of spit and mucus that trail from the head of a cock when a gagger's mouth is pulled back and off the cock. One fetish includes making the giver vomit as well.

Biting

I love kissing and biting. Gently, sweetly, firmly, menacingly. I love to bite the tongue, the lips—both inside and outside. I love to run my open mouth against the sides and top of my lover's head—teeth pressing firm and solid. I love to bite the cheeks and neck, back, calves, feet—anything, everything—forcing my lover to wonder, shuddering, what I might do next. I love to find a wide part of flesh, and slowly close my lips and mouth and press my teeth deep, not hard enough to break skin—but just enough to leave my mark.

You'd think our mouths only had tongues, lips, and gums when it comes to sex. Let's change that.

Teeth are toys you carry with you all the time. Nipping, nibbling, teeth dragging, and lots of variations of biting can be part of your sex vocabulary. Hold off on the slurping, lip smacking, or steady chewing—trust me, not so sexy. As with all other techniques I've discussed, start gently. The more you warm up someone's flesh, the longer and perhaps deeper they will be able to go. The longer you maintain the bite, the more pain is registered. The smaller the area of skin that is pressed between the teeth, the more painful it is. Givers, be random yet conscious of what, where, and how you bite. Receivers: Ask your lover to bite you. Pay attention to how much you can receive and where it feels best, and don't be bashful about telling your partner when something feels wonderful or horrid.

Biting can mark or break the skin, leaving teeth marks and bruises. Unless you and your partner are fluid-bonded—you are aware of each other's HIV and STI test results and agree to exchange bodily fluids—don't draw blood. This isn't about vampirism (though that's a sexy fetish, for sure). Any STI that can be transmitted through blood can be transferred through biting. Even kissing carries risks of infection, including hepatitis A, hepatitis B, and herpes.

It's pretty common for biting and sucking to go together, aka biting with hickeys. Check in about marks before or during your sex tumble; a few simple words ("Are marks okay?") usually will do the trick. But remember, once the adrenalin and endorphins kick in, it's easy to get "sex-stupid" and say yes to everything. Have the "marks" chat before or early in the game. If you don't know that marks are okay, avoid leaving them. And, right, there are no guarantees. Just make sure either that your partner doesn't have that family beach reunion tomorrow or that he wants to wear the memory of your chompers with pride.

Full-mouth biting is sensuous personified. Very light can tickle, very heavy can be excruciating. Find meaty or soft spots like arms, breasts, pecs, the back of the neck, and the ass. Use extra awareness and caution with the side of the neck (those tendons can hurt in that bad way), taut muscles, bone, the genitals, the inner thighs, and the face.

Finally, biting doesn't have to hurt but it can—a lot. Each of us has a different pain threshold. Watch your partner, and if it is your wont, play on the edge of what she can take. If she says stop, you stop. Use a safeword. Here are some ideas:

- Drag your teeth across the shoulder, thigh, belly, back, breast, top of head (hair and all), butt. Vary the speed and depth of the drag.

- Bite slowly and repeatedly in the same place, building tension and depth.

- Open your mouth wide and press it against the meaty flesh of your choice (back, belly, ass). Slowly sink your teeth in. Close your mouth slowly and steadily, pressing, gripping, and holding. You can let off the pressure, but don't release the bite. You can also gently shake your head, as a lion shakes its kill. Your partner will swoon, ache, throb, squirm. Your goal isn't necessarily to inflict pain but to cause such out-of-the-ordinary, exquisite sensations that his head begins to pop off.

- Some people love biting genitals or having theirs bitten; others might haul off and smack you one or call you a cab, so go lightly at first. The labia, balls, and shaft of the penis are very sensitive; even more sensitive are the clitoris and the head of the penis. Use your front teeth and gently press on any of these tender bits of flesh, not fully closing. Then close and release. Or while holding this tender flesh between your teeth, run or flick your tongue against your lucky victim.

Rough Hand Sex

There are many things we get to do with our hands when getting rough during sex: penetrate, pinch, slap, punch, flick, stroke, scratch, rub, smack, knead, press, and so on. Like your teeth, your hands are always with you and can be two of the most versatile sex toys (along with that other gorgeous one throbbing in your skull). You can use your fingers and hands for vaginal and anal penetration, fisting, hand jobs, and more. These are just a few ways to include your fingers and hands in sex. Using latex or nonlatex gloves and lube are sure ways to make any kind of penetration less susceptible to infection and disease transmission, and will do wonders to give a smooth ride to the receiver.

Set the stage by talking about your intentions before you get busy. Check in verbally with simple words, without cockiness or worry: "I want to fuck you hard with my hand, okay? It's so okay to say no, my precious slut." Once you get the go-ahead, don't stop paying attention to your lover, but *now*, take what you want. Watch and listen to your lover's reactions.

For vaginal penetration, start slowly, watching and listening to your lover. (Use lube as needed.) Keep checking in periodically. Once her body is as full or almost as full as is comfortable, move your fingers in and out, building speed and intensity. Go slowly, just don't let go of the intensity—the feeling of doggedness and hunger on your part can be a huge turn-on for your partner. You can fuck long, deep, and hard or short, fast, and hard—combine these in various ways. Curl your fingers toward the navel and stimulate the G-spot. With one hand penetrating the vagina, the other hand is free to cause other delicious trouble—choking, slapping, squeezing breasts and nipples. Throw in some mouth action too: sucking or biting her belly, breasts, and cunt. Slowly increase the intensity and speed of your thrusts. (Thrusting intensity and speed are separate things.) Remember, if you're fucking a vagina, pounding the cervix (located at the back of the vagina) can be a painful experience. Be ready to shift positions if your partner tells you it hurts.

When fucking your partner's ass with your hand—even if you're "raping" them—you *must* use lube. Spit does not count—end of story. The ass cannot make its own lubrication, and if not treated properly the thin skin of the rectum can tear easily, making both receiver and giver susceptible to bacteria and STIs. Plus, no lube equals bad pain. Start slowly with one or two fingers or a small toy with a condom on it, and build larger as his body allows. Once his body is as full or almost as full as is comfortable, move your fingers in and out, building speed and intensity. Tell him that you own that hole. You can fuck long, deep, and hard or short, fast, and hard. The common element is hard—this is rough sex, after all. Curl your fingers toward the navel and stimulate the G-spot or the P-spot (prostate).

And receivers of anal sex? You think just because you like rough sex your ass is supposed to hurt and feel ripped open? No—really no. Don't use poppers or numbing creams—if it hurts, tell your partner to slow down or stop. Bad pain sucks. It also makes you "ass shy" for future anal romps. Remember, rough sex means *more* communication and negotiation—not less. Tell him his junk is too damned big—and he should take it up his own damned ass if he thinks it's so damned easy.

Fingers and Mouth Play
Putting your fingers in someone's mouth can be unspeakably sexy. It's also a great way to objectify someone and make them feel deliciously used by you for your sexual gratification. Bend two or three fingers into her mouth, press your thumb onto her chin or under her jaw, and grab hold. Move her head to the position you want it—a better angle to kiss you, to put your nipple, cock, or cunt in her mouth, to slap her face, etc. Have him suck your fingers as if they were your cock. Instruct him to open his mouth and keep it open. Insert two, three, four, or even five fingers into the waiting mouth and "fuck" his face with your hand. Try this in a variety of positions. While penetrating her from behind with dildo and harness or penis, pull her hair by the roots to arch her back, bringing her head toward you. Insert your hand and fuck her face this way. Be sure you judge how deep you want your fingers to go—the head tipped back makes for a more narrow space in her throat; if gagging is not your and her thing, be careful to not push too hard or deep.

Slapping

Being on the receiving end of slapping makes me feel very, very small and submissive. It is the single fastest way to get me into a bottom head space. I get very quiet, inside and out. At the same time, whether it's because I'm wired this way or because I now associate the two activities (slapping and sex), I get aroused.

—MANDY

Let's talk about slapping, face slapping, and punching. It's important to know where it's safe to hit someone's body. (Have I mentioned consent recently? Here is your reminder that you need consent in order for any of this *not* to be abusive. Explicit, noncoerced consent.) Check out Illustration 9.1: Where to strike. All the places marked 1 and 2 are perfect for slapping. Places marked 3 should not be hit.

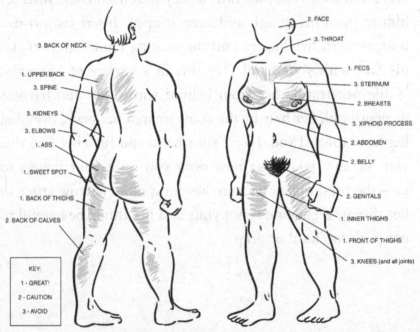

Illustration 9.1. Where to strike

There are three basic kinds of slaps: cupped hand, open/flat hand, and fingertips only.

Cupped-Hand Slap

Your hand is extended, fingers together, slightly bent. When the hand connects with the skin, it makes a hollow sound. This is the least stingy of the three types of slaps; it's a great one for beginners, for warm-up, and for anywhere on the body (including genitals).

Open/Flat-Hand Slap

The hand is positioned just as the name suggests. Use this slap everywhere that's safe to strike, with varying amounts of intensity and depth. You don't have to haul off and slap somebody silly simply because you want to play rough. Repetitive, gentle slapping—especially on sensitive areas—can feel remarkable. Light slaps feel sharp and stingy, while heavy ones will leave a tingling, burning sensation for some time after the hand is removed. This slap is great for butt, face, belly, chest, and thighs, and lightly on genitals.

Fingertip Slap

Ow! This is a mean one. Imagine swatting away the hand reaching for your last cookie, using your fingertips to connect with the offending hand or arm and then pulling off quickly. That's this one. Can be used with care anywhere on your lover's body to make it sting.

Face Slapping

Perhaps you want to slap someone's face. Or have yours slapped. You're in great company. Face slapping can change the direction and intensity of a scene like nothing else, allowing the one who is slapping to feel turned on and powerful over his lover, and the one receiving the slap to feel intense intimacy, "put in his place," made to feel small, loved, humiliated, turned on, quiet, woken up—a million amazing things. Face slapping can also bring up immediate, unexpected emotional responses like rage, tears, or panic.

Unlike what we see in the movies, face slapping can really hurt; it can be disorienting and humiliating. If someone's past includes physical, verbal, or sexual abuse, whether in childhood or adulthood, face slapping may send them into a tailspin, making everyone feel pretty bad. Be sure to mention face slapping specifically when you and your partner discuss what works and doesn't work for you. Even if you are already getting busy, check in first before you slap someone's face. Holding his head, show him your hand and ask, "Yes?" Wait for a response before you continue. This goes for people who have been lovers for a while too—today might have been a tough day for her, and face slapping will be too much to deal with. If your partner has TMJ (a chronic inflammation of the jaw) or other jaw issues, don't do this. Avoid the cheek and jawbones, eyes, and ears. You might want to take off those glasses too.

When you have your partner's consent, support the right side of her head with your left hand (opposite for lefties). Spread your fingers apart so that the ear is not pressed between your

> ## FACE SLAPPING IDEAS
>
> - She's on her knees sucking your cock. Holding the left side of her head and steadying her jaw, slap her face. Remember, her teeth are very close to your sensitive cock; by steadying her jaw, you minimize risk of accidental bites (or payback bites!). You can also pull her mouth off your cock, slap her, and then put her right back where you both want her.
>
> - Instead of using your hand to support his head, press one side of his face onto a soft or firm surface. This is great for getting busy with the other hand. Use great caution here, though: a wall or floor, even the bed or a pillow, doesn't have the give that your other hand would have. A slap is felt more intensely in these positions.
>
> - Want to up the ante? Once you've established that face slapping is a go, try slapping her without holding the side of her head. Be careful that her head does not snap back or to the side. Try a few backhand slaps as well.

fingers and her head. Supporting the head like this prevents the head and neck from being jerked suddenly and damaging to the neck. It's also a great way to get eye contact with your lover: a perfect moment for the giver to "own" the moment, keeping calm and attitudinally tall. Watch as that energy transfers through your hands and eyes to your partner and back again—it's electrifying and sexy, and it can be hugely moving. With your right hand, place your *fingers* (not palm) on the fleshy part of her cheek. Don't include her jaw, eye, or ear. When you're learning this technique it's easy to miss the target, so do a slow trial run. Pull your hand back and *place* it on her cheek. Start slowly and lightly. After you deliver a slap or two, check in. Ask, "On a scale of one to ten, how hard was that?" This is a great way to discover what she wants as well as to gauge your strength. (It's a common complaint, especially of people who study martial arts, work out, or do a lot of manual labor, that it's difficult to know what too hard looks like.) This gets you two talking, as well.

Punching
There is something explicitly erotic to me about being punched, the flesh-on-flesh of it sends my mind into a place like nothing else does.

Punching is an aspect of rough sex that at first glance might freak you out, but punching during fucking is sexy, fun, and mighty, and something that tons of people are into. Gender, muscle power, and size are irrelevant—the playing field can be leveled by desire. It's certainly not just the domain of athletes or men: countless nonjock women—queer and straight, tough and tender—adore punching and getting punched as part of their sex. It builds and releases a deep, primal energy exchange between giver and receiver. It's incredibly intimate, especially face to face. It's verboten. It's fun and fierce. You get to feel "taller" in yourself and in the world. Both givers and receivers can push themselves like marathon runners, getting off on the release of their pent-up junk and feeling happy, whole, and high from the release of endorphins. They get to tap into their fierce animal selves, otherwise held captive by the daily confines of rules, assumptions, fears.

However, family and society teach that hitting between lovers is abuse; if you like to hit or be hit, you are mentally and emotionally unstable; boys are never supposed to hit girls; girls wouldn't want to hit boys; two girls hitting each other is funny—it's a catfight (or bad porn); two boys hitting each other is normal and has nothing to do with sex; trans people don't exist, so they don't even make it into the equation. *Forget all of it.* Really. Useless crap. The one thing to learn and remember: When there is *explicit consent*, the doors to boundless possibilities in sex swing wide open.

How to Punch

This isn't a street brawl or Gold's Gym; there is no boxing ring and there are no adversaries—you're both on the same team, with a common goal: joining together to make your sex unspeakably hot and raucous. Know your own strength—you're going for controlled *sensation* not a knockout. Build up slowly, see what turns on your partner. As I advised above, don't slap or punch when you're angry; this is not a substitute for resolving conflicts with love and respect.

Givers: Make a fist, thumb in front, outside. Use the flat part of your fingers or the side or back of your fist (or you can slightly lift your middle knuckle and make that the first point of contact), keeping the wrist firm but not locked. Do *not* use your full strength—especially when starting out. Stay aware of your body and your strength, and of how to place a punch as opposed to throwing one without care for where it lands. Remember too that what the receiver may want and what feels good to her today may be undesirable tomorrow, depending on her mood and physical health, including her menstrual cycle. Vary the depth and speed of punches; light, repetitive punches can build anticipation and allow the receiver to find the head space to go deeper and receive more.

Receivers: Don't clench up when receiving a punch. Breathe. If being punched on a certain part of your body doesn't turn you on, try another meaty muscled spot. Or say no, thank you. Don't give in to fear, or allow yourself to discover what might feel exquisite. Asking your partner to lighten up or shift position slightly is a sign of an engaged and passionate partner. Good for you.

You can punch anywhere on the body you can spank or slap. Areas good for punching: back (the meaty back/shoulder muscles), upper and inner thighs (inner is more sensitive), chest/pecs, side/upper arms, and ass. Areas you shouldn't punch: joints, spine, kidneys, bony protrusions, throat, neck, sternum, feet, hands, ears, and eyes. There are a multitude of opinions regarding whether or not it is safe to punch breasts. It has been said that punching breasts can cause cysts to develop or damage already existing cysts. The generally accepted guidelines are to punch the pectoral muscles, not the breasts or the sternum.

Bruising

Not all punching leads to bruising—not even close. But since everyone bruises differently, I'm including a few simple steps to take in case you bruise after an especially hot encounter. Some medications can cause people to bruise more easily, including blood thinners, antihistamines, and aspirin. Tylenol and Advil do not increase susceptibility to bruising. If you are concerned about visible bruises, apply ice to reduce possible swelling; after 24 to 48 hours you may switch to warm compresses. A cold shower may reduce bruising; a hot one can reactivate it later. (Some people get off on their sex bruises as memories of love or heat.) Bruising often takes hours or even days to appear.

It's common for the appearance of bruises to travel. Your *breast* may turn all sorts of rainbow colors but you are sure that only your *pecs* were punched. Generally this is not a problem and the bruises will fade. Using the herb arnica—available at most drugstores in a cream or gel or as an edible herb in pill form at health food stores—can help reduce the occurrence or persistence of bruising. You can take it before or after you play. If heavy impact is a big part of your scene, you might feel the next day as though you were hit by a Mack truck, or exhibit flu symptoms. Drink lots of water and keep an eye on the swelling.

Breath Play and Choking
He opened the door, shoved his way in, and pinned me by my throat against the smooth wall of the hallway. He kissed me so hard I thought he would bruise my mouth. I don't even

know what happened, but he made his mouth a seal that enveloped mine and then he held my nose closed with his other hand. That fear that makes me so crazy slipped over me and I could feel myself weaken in his grip. He decided when it was time for me to breathe—to take air; he let the seal between our lips loosen for only a moment and then owned my breath all over again. God, I loved it.

Controlling someone's breath with your hand or mouth (breath play) is very intimate and can be dangerous and scary as well. One way to do it is described above. Here are a few variations:

- Kiss your partner, making a seal over both mouth and nose. Breathe rhythmically. Soon you are each breathing the other's inhalations and exhalations.
- Place one hand over your partner's mouth and pinch her nostrils closed.
- Bite and suck with your mouth, play with his nipples and breasts with your free hand. Release the nostrils when it's time for him to breathe.

Breath play is quite prevalent in porn, and many people equate choking or strangulation with rough sex. But I'm going to tell you right now, there is *no way* to choke someone without huge risk of injury or possible death. There is abundant documentation of heart attacks, brain damage, seizures, and crushed larynxes—all these effects and more have been clearly linked to choking, strangulation, and other forms of controlling your own or another's breathing.

But since telling kids that abstinence is the best birth control hasn't done squat to reduce teenage pregnancy, let me tell you how to choke someone in a *safer* way. Notice that I don't say "safe"? There is no way to guarantee safety, folks—none.

Many people find choking during oral sex, intercourse, or kissing a huge turn-on. It heightens sensations, causes head rushes, and enhances the feeling of taking and being taken. One way to create the now-I'm-forced-and-helpless feeling of choking without choking is to wrap your hand around your partner's throat without any pressure while you're fucking. Although your hand may cover the larynx, do not press against it—it's far too fragile and can be crushed by too much pressure. Once again, as in spanking and face slapping, being ever aware of the placement, strength, and pressure of your hands is vital. Place your thumb and forefinger on either side of the throat under the jaw, back toward the ears. Press into the throat and up toward the ears and squeeze your fingers against the carotid arteries, reducing blood flow to the brain.

Pressing (not slamming) your partner's head into a pillow or against the wall gives you more leverage—but might make him pass out. Everyone's body has a shutoff valve to protect itself, but because each person's threshold is different, there is no way to know when someone might pass out. Passing out is enormously dangerous: there's no way to recover those brain cells that were killed, and he could have a heart attack or a stroke. If you see his eyes rolling back in his head, stop. Learn everything you can about breath play before you try it on anyone. I recommend you attend a class at a BDSM event taught by a reputable teacher.

BRUTAL AFFECTION AFTERCARE

When you play rough, your body can get marked up. You can have surface or deep bruising, redness of the skin, scrapes, and even internal bruising (cervix, pelvic bone, inside of mouth). Always check in with your partner before doing something that might leave a mark. And remember that everyone's skin is different—some people bruise, mark, and scar more easily than others. I remember, the first time I played rough with a lover, I was careful about how I slapped her face, but bam! She got a black eye. I felt pretty rotten, but my lover thought it looked tough. Lucky for me, tough was good. Another time, I thought I kneed my partner with careful force between his butt cheeks as he stood, but I was wrong. He had to go to several extra chiropractic visits for a bruised coccyx (tailbone). Experience and consent were present in both situations, and, well, shit happens.

The emotional risks of this kind of sex play are even more unpredictable. Depending on one's history of abuse or trauma, sex in general can bring up big emotions—often taking us by surprise. Many people report weeping at or immediately following orgasm. This doesn't mean something horrible happened—just a huge swell of emotions that came unplugged with the release of tension and chemicals in the muscles and brain. Bring in power play, primal responses, physical roughness—regardless of consent being clearly

IDEAS, POSITIONS, AND PLACES

- Missionary never felt so good. He's fucking you hard as you lie on your back: you pound on his back with your fists.
- You're sitting on top straddling your lover: punch the pecs (avoid breasts and sternum).
- While spanking him, throw in a few punches—the thudding sensation is a perfect counterbalance to the sting of the slap.
- Restrain by rope, pallet wrap, or leather restraints. (When someone is retrained, he is unable to move with the punch and therefore absorbs the full power behind it—accommodate as needed.)
- Try it on the floor, in a chair, or standing against a wall in a hall, alley, bathroom, hotel room, pool.
- Try it with your partner's legs spread/tied open—fuck her cunt while you punch her chest.
- Bend him over a couch or bed—fuck his ass, punch his back, ass, and upper thighs.
- Remember, punching is one more thrilling ingredient to make your sex a magnificent feast.

given—and the stakes get higher, the possible responses bigger. Trusting your partner is key. If you know you might respond negatively to a particular activity, warn your partner away from doing it, or tell her what might happen and what she should do in response. One more great reason to have a safeword or gesture.

Even after many years of understanding and coming to terms with my childhood abuse, I still have unexpected responses during sex; sometimes I get scared and lose track of where I am or who I'm with. Moreover, because my abuse started preverbally, I sometimes lose the ability to speak my needs in these moments. Being aware of this and telling my lovers about it when we're talking about our desires and needs allows us to establish supportive strategies if something comes up. Taking care of myself sets another brick into the foundation of trust and safety we build. Couple that with articulated desire and consent? Stand back for Richter-scale sex.

YOU'RE A GREAT LOVER. NOW GET BETTER.

Sex is about the journey, not the arrival. It's a verb, not a noun. It requires bravery and compassion for yourself and your lover. Remember that laughing can save a far too serious scene or sex that's threatening to become boring. If something is funny—you can't walk with those new 10-inch stilettos you just got, or the phone rings in the middle of the deserted-island fantasy you both created—laugh. Just make sure you're laughing *with* your partner, please.

And don't forget to breathe! Fear, pain, anger, frustration—these are just a few reasons why we forget to breathe. Yes, forget. When we are so focused on taking the sexy hard stuff being doled out to us, it's easy to hold our breath. Givers, if you notice your lover holding his breath, remind him to breathe. If you are playing with power, you can say, "Give me your breath." Perhaps it's corny, but it works. Breathing allows much deeper sensuality, connection, and experience. And you givers, if you're not breathing, you're not in your body enough to keep you and your lover safe and turned on.

Rough sex is far more than simply banging away on

someone. Rough sex is taking and being taken. Ravaging and being ravaged. Pushing and being pushed. Letting go and letting go. Rough sex is an attitude. It's a journey. And it's truly astounding. Talk. Fuck. Play. Risk. Love. Laugh. Respect.

Go get 'em, tiger. And don't forget the lube.

Endnotes

1   Chasing the Jersey, "Why I Sleep With Athletes And Why You Should, Too," December 24, 2010, http://www.sportsgrid.comnfl/chasing-the-jersey-why-i-sleep-with-athletes-and-why-you-should-too/.

CHAPTER 10

BUTTHOLE BLISS: THE INS AND OUTS OF ANAL FISTING

PATRICK CALIFIA

Anal fisting (or handballing) is one of the most extreme sexual acts that one person can allow another to do to his or her body. In fact, some so-called experts still deny that it's even physically possible. Ha! What do they know? I have been there and done that with more people than you've probably had sex with in your whole life. And so have happy hosts of other sexual gourmets. So I'm here to tell you it can be done (and how). Putting your whole hand up somebody else's butt is an exhilarating experience. When you can feel those hot, greasy membranes close around your wrist and forearm, and your partner's heartbeat feels as if it is literally in the palm of your hand, there is nothing more intimate. You are sharing an erotic space that has the potential to become a temple both sacred and profane. Few other things can equal the rush. Unless, of course, you're the one who is getting handballed. Oh, yeah, I almost forgot that part.

But anal fisting is also one of the most potentially dangerous things a bottom can ask a top to do. There is no room here for getting it almost right. You need to be able to demand perfection of yourself and your partner. Ironically and paradoxically, before you can pig out, you have to have acquired a sort of exotic discipline that never lets up. Nine-tenths of fisting has nothing to do with the act itself, but with the preparation. Something that may look depraved and even brutal is actually as formal as any high holy day ritual. Are you washed in the blood of the lamb? Try some Crisco instead. Because we don't want any blood here, or even any pain.

Handballing is, on one level, just another form of fucking. Penetration given and received is about as vanilla as it gets. This is why some who fly the red hanky feel that their fetish has little or nothing to do with BDSM. Being around people who are getting noisily spanked and whipped and are screaming to the rhythm of the cane can be too distracting for some degenerates who enjoy heavy anal play. They prefer to keep these activities away from leathersex. If they are going to play in a group, it will be a group of other handballers, with the appropriate background music: a lot of bass, and the moans and groans of others whose asses are being judiciously tormented.

In fact, the notorious San Francisco fisting club The Catacombs was founded by Steve McEachern in part because his brothers in the Fist Fuckers of America (FFA) objected to his love of bondage, flagellation, and other kinkiness. If pain turns you on, a pair of nipple clamps or a slap or 12 on the butt might be the foreplay you need to open up and take it good. In my opinion, that's more about how the individual is wired than any kind of moral claim that one sort of sex might have to being better than another.

But making a distinction is still useful because of what is required to do fisting safely. In some ways, I would rather do handballing with an individual who is not a masochist, because they are more likely to understand that I don't want them putting up with any anal or rectal pain. I'm sadistic as hell, but this is one sex act that I want to take place with as little discomfort as possible. Outright pain is a sign that something is going very wrong! Things never ought to get to that point. But a compliant bottom who is grooving on getting hurt can keep his or her mouth shut until injury may occur. Which is my worst nightmare.

Anal fisting is near the end of the line in a long series of warm-up acts of sodomy. The first time somebody rubs a little spit on the outside of your asshole and you feel yourself shiver, who knows if that's where you are headed? Because there's no wrong or right place to go with a love of anal sex; rimming is no more or less wonderful than sitting on a dildo that's 12 inches around. The point with all forms of sex is to make each other feel good. If all you like is vanilla, there's no point to engaging in other acts just to make yourself look cool. Within the realm of what we sometimes dismiss as vanilla is enough wisdom and sensuality to confound the angels. There's good information about anal sex technique in books devoted to the subject, so I will just add a couple of my personal parameters.

The first and most important is, you will enjoy anal sex a lot more if you can make a contract with your butt that you will never allow it to be hurt. You don't have to get fucked in a hurry to prove that you are worthwhile or fun. Slow the fuck down and relish what you are doing.

The same dictum goes for tops. Knowing how to handball is based on a bunch of Assplay 101 seminars. You need to have sensitive hands that can tell when that little muscle is aching to be opened up, and when it's just aching. The strong muscles in your forearm are meant to keep the ride going for a long time—not to bully your way past some imaginary doorkeeper. I like to tell the bottom that what we are doing is teasing their asshole and making it so hungry that it's going to start sucking things up, opening up and drawing what it craves into itself. I am just going to hold still and let him or her show me how much they need. (Of course this is a lie; I can't really hold still for very long. Even if I got my ADHD meds.) But there are many motions that arouse the anus other than simple thrusting. Stroking, vibrating, and tickling, plus smoothing out the big muscles around the opening—these are all helpful to aid relaxation, dilation, arousal, and release.

PREPARATION

Preparation for a fisting scene begins about 48 hours before the date. This is because most fisters want the rectum and colon to be cleaned out before play begins. Going on a diet of soft foods or liquids that pass quickly through your body is step one. Six to eight hours before the date itself, you can start with a series of enemas that will keep your bowel free from obstruction. Use tepid water. Water that is too cold will cause cramping, and you don't want water that is too hot, for obvious reasons. Many fisters get tired of filling up and emptying those bags you buy at the drugstore, and have a hose installed on their shower. A nozzle should ideally be used by one person only. If it has to be shared, soak it in a 10% bleach solution, but be aware that this may not kill hepatitis B or C. Using the hoses at a club is a recipe for getting a sexually transmitted infection (STI), so don't do it. If you are a visitor from out of town, resign yourself to buying an enema bag at a local pharmacy and using it repeatedly.

How long does it take to clean out? This varies so much from one individual to another that I don't know how to answer this question. Your diet as well as your anatomy and the level of control you have over it are important factors. Some are lucky enough to be able to take water in and eliminate it smoothly. Others needs to wait around, read the newspaper, take a walk, etc., before the water will drop. Getting rid of all the water is as important as getting rid of all the poo. It's considered extremely rude to hit your top in the face with a wave of unclean aqua. Give yourself enough time to feel really prepared. Rushing it will just make douching, as it's known, feel uncomfortable. Creating a lot of cramping with hasty enemas may make it harder for your butt to relax during handballing.

Douching is necessary for three reasons. One: Most of the people who like ass play do not, oddly enough, like shit. Two: Even a partially full bowel can cause contractions that make penetration painful. Three: Feces with a gritty texture should not be ground against the delicate lining of your rectum and lower bowel. People who enjoy scat have their own sets of techniques, mores, and safety precautions that are beyond the scope of this article.

The top also ought to spend a similar amount of time in preparation. Do some yoga, meditate, journal, do what you need to do to put yourself in a good frame of mind, with lots of energy. Don't show up with a cold or a rotten attitude. You will be using your body just as much as your partner uses theirs, so pay attention to your own well-being. Eat some protein before you play so you don't get a big crash in your blood sugar. Groom your hands. Remove every sharp cuticle and trace of fingernail. Do this even if you are going to be wearing gloves! The lining of the rectum is not very thick; puncturing it can have dire consequences in terms of infection and bleeding. So if the tip of your glove breaks, for any reason, make sure that there is nothing abrasive on your fingertip that can cause harm. This also alters your hands and turns them into sexual symbols with the potency of genitals.

Once you and your partner are together, do whatever the two of you enjoy to get turned on. There's no rule that says you have to throw yourself into a sling in the first five minutes. Tops who like to get off may choose to have the bottom make them come before play, to take some of the edge off their nerves. Some bottoms find that an orgasm helps them to relax. For others, coming just makes them lose interest in any more sex.

The topic of drugs and alcohol inevitably comes up during

a discussion of preparing for the main act. If you've read any leather community history, you will know that drugs used to be a very big part of the gay men's fisting scene. In fact, doing fisting without them was practically unheard of. MDA was a popular relaxant then, but people also drank alcohol, popped Quaaludes, did crystal meth, dropped acid, snorted coke, swallowed a variety of prescription sedatives and muscle relaxers, and came up with other unique and sometimes scary combinations. And, of course, the brown bottles of amyl nitrate (or after that became illegal, butyl nitrate) were ubiquitous.

I've been clean and sober for nearly 20 years, but I can't lie to you: being intoxicated did help people relax, shed their inhibitions, and dilate their orifices. But the high level of drug use also led to addiction (which I define as repeatedly trying to get high when it stopped being fun a long time ago), overdoses, unwise selection of partners, imprecise communication, blunted pain, overuse of the back door, and a lot of depressed and sore mornings after spent with one ice bag on the forehead and another between the buttocks.

If you are a pervert and an addict in recovery, you have no choice but to learn how to enjoy your wicked ways without the use of mind-altering substances. This probably deserves its own chapter or even a book. But if you are not an addict, I see nothing wrong with one drink (and I do mean one). There are many people who would disagree with me. The politically correct injunction is not to drink or use any drugs when you play. This may be an ideal, but it's not the way many people actually have sex. I think we are doing poor sex education if we don't look at how erotic behavior actually takes place, and offer people interventions that are reasonable. If you don't know your own body well enough to understand what kind of psychotropic substances you can ingest without harm, you are an arrogant novice or willfully ignorant, and nothing I can say will help you. Unfortunately, I still see a lot of us engaging in self-harm, perhaps because we feel guilty about our deviant sex lives, or we've got a lot of baggage from fucked-up families of origin, or perhaps our friends are giving us stupid advice and pressuring us to do as they do. I want all of us to have scads of fun and love in our lives with as little damage as possible. Be careful of your precious self. If you need to get injured, emotionally obliterated, or killed to fulfill a wrongheaded, romantic idea of your own doomed specialness, it's not as if you won't be able to find a bunch of villains who will oblige you. Dammit.

Assuming you are a sensible person who has managed to line up an opportunity to misbehave, you can maximize your chances of a good experience by paying some attention to the environment where you meet. Some of us like to get our freak on at group sex events. If you've got access to that luxury, well and good. Hopefully the space will be clean and unlikely to draw the wrath of the vice squad by doing stupid things like admitting minors. A good sound system and the above-mentioned music help a lot as well. If you are playing in private, setting the mood doesn't have to mean constructing your own dungeon in a spare bedroom. Just clean up the room you are going to use, get rid of the dog bed and pictures of Grandma, and create a play surface. One solution is to cover the bed with a plastic sheet and then put something with a nicer texture on top of it. Some folks have invested in portable stands and slings. Other accessories include a couple of stacks of trick towels, some squeeze bottles of water, a large supply of lube, and any toys you might want to include in your Voyage to the Center of the Earth. Useful toys include vibrators, ass plugs and dildos, tit clamps, bondage restraints, genital whips, or cock rings. Don't forget condoms (to keep the toys clean) and gloves.

One of the most important items on this list is the lubricant. The classic of the 1970s and 1980s was, of course, Crisco. You knew you were with a cheap date if he showed up with generic vegetable shortening. When the AIDS epidemic got under way, the use of water-based lubricant became important for other types of sex, because oil can weaken the latex in condoms. Some fisters will swear that water-based lube is not thick enough and doesn't last long enough to make for a friction-free ride. I've seen recipes for mixing water-based lube with shortening, which allegedly gives you a product you can wash out of the sheets. (Don't count on it.) With experimentation, you will come up with your own answer. But I'd like to point out that you can use the thicker, longer-lasting grease if you are not going to need safer-sex protection later on. If you aren't going to be using condoms to contain sperms-and-germs, and if you are using nonlatex gloves, oil-based lube won't be dangerous. Keep in mind that the grease is going to linger in your tail for a few days, so think about what your sex life is going to include after the current date.

Remember that lubricant can be a source of disease transmission. If you have a big container of it, put some in smaller containers that can be discarded after play is done. Some people use paper cups; squeeze bottles or pumps are also handy. Just make sure that any lube you've touched is never used with another partner. Even if you are both healthy, the bacteria and other microorganisms from the colon could make somebody else sick.

Keep the room nice and warm. Cold makes muscles tense up, and your asshole is a muscle. For most of us, decent music is also very erotic and helpful during tough bits of the play. It can lift the mood and strengthen the bond between players during nonverbal moments. Keep up with what's current in the clubs and make your own tapes or buy good ones. Think of it as lubricant for your ears.

What is the best way to position your bodies? Slings became popular because they created a weightless sensation, and the top could move one back and forth, like the rocking of a cradle. But many people don't like them. It can be hard to make a good pillow for a sling, and who can ignore a crick in the neck, no matter how loud their prostate is humming? Some bottoms do better if they can get up on their hands and knees. I think it's good to keep the option of changing positions, since moving the whole body will also affect the target orifice.

JOURNEY TO BLISS

When you are facing the bottom, with the bottom on their back, you probably want to make the initial approach with your left hand: the rectum naturally bends the same way your wrist will bend. Apply some lube to the outer opening and massage it in. Use fingers or toys to gradually expand the opening. You actually want to get lubricant inside the rectum. That's tricky until the asshole begins to gape a bit, and you can shove some in on your fingertips. You can hook one finger around the lip of the anal orifice, stretch it a bit, and use your other hand to tuck a gob of lube past the ring of muscle. If you are already inside and it feels like you need more lube, carefully remove your hand, fill up your palm, and go back in. Then squeeze your hand to release the lube.

Should you talk to the bottom or let them go off on their own mental trip? I prefer partners who stay connected to me while we play. I need to check in with them about what feels good and what does not, how fast or deep I should go—so I want that channel to stay open. I recommend not letting the two of you get too far apart. If you can maintain communication nonverbally, through body movement and eye contact, that's fine—but it's also not too common. It's okay for the top to ask, "Are you groaning because you want more, or are you having trouble?" Reassure the bottom that it is okay to ask for a break, more lube, less lube, tit work, genital stimulation, etc. Also let them know that the play is not goal-oriented. If you don't get your whole hand inside them, that's okay. (And they won't believe you unless that's true, so curb your enthusiasm.)

Talking can be a way to take control of the bottom's internal experience. By tweaking his or her emotions, you can also make their body give sway. Fisting can have dozens of different meanings in the context of the relationship between top and bottom. It is the top's job to identify, name, and sell that meaning. "You're doing this because you belong to me. It's the ultimate way of giving me ownership over your body." "I want to get you higher than you've ever been before. You know that nobody can make you feel the way that I can make you feel." "You're a dirty little piggy. You can never get enough. Now everybody is going to know what an utter whore you are. See how much you need this?" "I'm touching you because I love you. Every time I push into your body, I'm pushing my love into you. And when you respond and give me what I want, I know that you love me too, because that energy hits me right in the heart. Feel that? Feel how much I love you?"

Remember that there are two bodies present. You can take a break and get sucked off, sixty-nine, do some bondage and flagellation, put on a hood or blindfold, trade back rubs, masturbate, or do anything else you both enjoy. I do not recommend doing play piercing or any other play that breaks the skin during fisting. Sweat and lubricant will be flying everywhere, carrying little travelers, and you don't want butt germs to enter the bloodstream.

As the butthole opens up, the top will feel some tension around the largest part of the hand. It takes experience to know when you should ignore it and go forward or wait for more dilation. The bottom's opinion ought to prevail. Use your fingertips to stroke the tissue inside the opening. Keep your hand pointed, folded up as small as possible, with the thumb tucked into the palm. You may approach this point of tension, back off, then work up to it again several times before you slide inside. Use your breaks to drink some water and make out. (Please don't tell me you are going to turn someone into your sock puppet but you won't kiss them!) When someone is learning how to get fisted, they may play without being completely penetrated for quite a while before their body learns to trust that these strange sensations are okay, and relaxes. Remember your prime directive: The Asshole Must Feel No Pain!

If you are lucky enough to be admitted, let the shape of the bowel direct the curve of your hand and wrist. Fisting is safest when you don't go any deeper than your wrist. Just sit where you are for a while, and let the bottom's body settle down. They may shake all over, cry out, and even cry. It's intense. You are in a very sensitive area, so you don't have to do a lot to create a big reaction. When you do start to move, keep it small. Make little circles. Gently open your hand a fraction of an inch, then close it again. Wiggle your fingertips. See what the response is to each of these gestures. If a prostate is available, a little extra pressure in that area can be sexy. But few men enjoy having the prostate hammered, so don't overdo it.

If there is enough wiggle room, get the fingertips of your other hand into heaven. This can help to introduce more lubricant. Also, some people enjoy a slow in-and-out in which you trade hands, one slipping past the other. Rotating your hand from side to side can also feel good. Eventually, you may be able to use the traditional in-and-out motion with one hand.

Having something that big inside your body usually changes the sexual response cycle. For example, guys may not get erections even if they feel very excited. Sometimes stimulating the penis or clitoris or vagina can help open the butthole up. But sometimes these sensations are too much, and don't have the desired effect. This can change from session to session. Often, people wind up focusing on the rush they are getting from the anal play. If they have a genital orgasm, it may come at the very end of the play. Fisting can sometimes make people piss. Get your next trick towel out, mop up, and proceed apace. It's a way of letting go, expanding emotional horizons, and releasing inhibitions. It can also feel grand. Don't make people wrong for an experience they can't prevent. Go with the flow. Literally.

From time to time, it is normal for the stimulated bowel to generate waves of contractions. Small ones can be ignored. Just hold still until it's over. But if you feel your hand being pushed out, let the body do what it needs to do. The feeling of having the hand expelled can be as pleasurable as being filled up. The anus is stretched no matter what direction you are going in. Engage in another activity or take a break until the bottom feels ready to get plugged again.

The bottom's physical challenge in a fisting scene is obvious. The top is also running a marathon, and perhaps those challenges need to be explained. The top will be putting out a lot of emotional energy through minute concentration and attention to detail. This is a lot of responsibility, and that affects an ethical person. It's also a huge ego rush. The top will probably be in uncomfortable positions for extended periods of time. If your nose itches or you have sweat in your eyes, your hands may not be clean enough to safely address the problem. (Have a clean bandana with the towels.) Your hand or arms can fall asleep. Your back can hurt. You may feel sleepy or get bored. Let's acknowledge that you are touching somebody else a lot, and for most of that time, no one is touching you, so you can experience alienation from your own body. The experienced fisting top learns how to minutely adjust position so blood can flow back into the feet or arms. With practice comes greater stamina.

You also learn when a cry for mercy actually means "I need just a little more to be able to get off"; when to call the opening in question a pussy or start narrating a fantasy about giving birth; when to shut the fuck up; and how to bring somebody down from the heights.

The orgasm is a marker for the end of a vanilla sex scene. Given the altered nature of the body during fisting, there may not be a single big explosion. Nevertheless, you can't do this forever, although it may sometimes feel as if you have created the perfect perpetual motion machine, a piston drilling for oil distilled from the Shadow itself. Sometimes the bottom will sense that they are through and signal that they need to stop. Sometimes the top needs to decide they can't continue, and inform the bottom that they are running out of steam and need to start coming back down to earth.

The process of extracting your hand can sometimes take as long as getting in. This isn't common, but you need to be aware that you don't just yank your hand out, wipe it off, and point the way to your door. Use the index finger of your other hand to open the asshole a bit, in case a seal has developed. You'll feel a release of air and can safely continue pulling back. Rotate your hand and verbally encourage the bottom to help you. Sometimes if they take a deep breath and gently bear down, you'll be smoothly expelled.

There are other ways to do fisting than what I've described

above. Some people enter the body past the wrist. There are also people who like punch-fucking, a rough and quick form of penetration. I am dubious about the safety of these activities. If you are going to do them, try to find an experienced person who understands the risks and can tell you how to minimize them. Where is the line between enough and too much? Every self-aware person has to confront that question and do their own experiments. My answer probably won't fit everyone else.

AFTERCARE AND SAFETY

If you still like each other afterward (you will probably like each other more), you can cuddle, say sweet things, and drink more water. Then it may be time to have a snack and go to sleep. But the top has usually built up quite a head of steam during this process. He or she needs some attention. The specific nature of the top's reward ought to be spelled out in advance. If you don't want to get off with the bottom's help, go home and treat yourself to a mean, slow session of jerking off, or find another warm body to do you. If tops ignore their own physical needs, they will eventually start to pull away from a specific partner or the technique that is perceived as draining and frustrating.

Forgive me for getting into the creaky old time machine once more, but I want to point out that fisting used to be a pitch-and-catch activity. There were almost no guys who topped exclusively, or men who did nothing but spread their legs and take it. It was understood that everybody was there to get fucked. Nobody with any common sense would trust their asshole to a man who hadn't experienced fisting himself. There was no shame in getting fisted. In fact, the more you could take, the more macho you were, in an odd way. This was in direct contrast to the SM community's more strictly segregated and formal roles.

Unfortunately, the brotherhood of butt worship has been subsumed into BDSM culture, for the most part, and that has meant a greater polarization between tops and bottoms. This isn't necessarily a bad thing. Those high-and-mighty deities of leather with their perfect boots have got their own appeal. And the tops aren't bad either. But I like to remind people that there are alternatives, different ways of looking at how these exchanges of erotic energy work, historical shifts and new possibilities for the future.

In conclusion I want to talk a little about sexual health and how to deal with an accident. During a fisting scene, it's extremely likely that the top will be exposed to whatever lurks within the bottom's bottom. This is why I encourage both parties to support their immune systems. A case of amoebas is hard to diagnose and unpleasant to treat. Hepatitis is more easily transmissible than HIV. Another potential problem is HPV, the human papillomavirus, which causes genital warts. Touching an infected part of someone's body and then touching yourself can pass it on. This is an extremely common virus, but some forms of it can dramatically increase a woman's risk of getting cervical cancer. There is a vaccine available for young women, and I urge everyone eligible to consider getting immunized. If you are going to have oral sex or penile penetration, then you may also have to worry about syphilis, gonorrhea, herpes, and the rest of the STIs. Be as healthy as you can be, use protection, and get tested regularly. If you come down with something, inform your partners, get treated, and don't pass it on. We can prove that we are a community by taking care of one another.

You can't rely on pain receptors to tell you if something has gone wrong deep inside the bowel, which is why the safest type of fisting is when you don't go any deeper than your wrist. Farther in than that the lining is much thinner. And if there is a problem, it will take longer for blood to show up, increasing the risk of a life-threatening issue.

Keep track of the color of your lube. Wipe some on a white towel from time to time. If it is turning pink, you are getting a little bit of blood, which means the lining is abraded. It's time to stop and find something else fun to do. If you see a spot of red blood, quit. Apply some ice. The bottom needs to monitor their belly and their body temperature. If they get a hard belly, experience internal pain, or start running a fever, it's time to call 911 and get to the emergency room. If you see a lot of blood, you're in big trouble. Apply pressure and call for help. This may mean that you need to keep your hand in place, inside the person, until medics arrive. Peritonitis takes hours to develop, but people bleed to death at top speed.

Hospitals can be scary places. Health workers like to think they have seen it all, but that doesn't mean they can't be sarcastic or judgmental toward people who have sex-related accidents. I don't know why those situations should be more embarrassing than a car accident, but reality is often unkind. In the ideal world, all of us would have insurance and primary care doctors who understood our sexuality. But we have to be prepared to cope with less than perfect emergency rooms. A top who abandons a bottom in this situation is a complete and total jerk. Stay with the person who is hurt. Advocate for them. You need the staff to understand that this is not a case of domestic violence. It was consenting sex that went wrong, and you are very, very sorry. If it looks as if they might report this to the police as a case of assault, call your lawyer. (You do have a lawyer, don't you?) There are no known cases of this happening, but who wants to be the exception?

Now you can see why I urge you to approach handballing with the greatest of respect. I have never to my knowledge hurt anybody I've played with, but I've also frequently refused to do things I felt were unsafe, even if my partner begged me to continue. Bodies are unpredictable things. If there is a weak spot in a partner's blood vessel or rectal lining, I could theoretically hurt them even if I was doing something I've safely done to others. Err on the side of caution.

Honestly, this game is not for every player. Some of us are disqualified just by virtue of our bodies. Hips or orifices refuse to stretch that much. Minds or hearts know it is not wise, but refuse to let go. Some of us might be able to go there, but we know that we can't deal with the consequences if an accident happens. If you don't have good medical care and access to legal protection, don't take risks that exceed your resources. I would offer the same advice to someone who liked to be catheterized, for example, or anyone who wanted to get pregnant, for that matter.

If such scary things could happen, why do people do handballing at all? Should we declare fisting off-limits for the Safe, Sane, and Consensual crowd? I'm not sure the question is even worth asking, because when people want something for purposes of arousal and physical delight, they will go to great lengths to do it, even if it is dangerous or forbidden. Sometimes forbidding something makes it more appealing. I believe it is better to give people a lot of information about the pros and cons of various sexual behaviors so they can decide for themselves.

Handballing is like modern dance, the feats of Hindu fakirs, or an ordeal that creates a shaman. People do it because it demands everything they've got. There is a high obtained from pushing your body to the limits and beyond, and in doing something extraordinary that most people can't even imagine. Giving up control of such a private and demeaned part of the body, allowing someone else to pleasure you and worship your butt, lifts centuries of culturally induced shame from our shoulders. It is a way of saying, I am different, I can do something amazing, I know a closely guarded secret. My life has magic in it.

Author's Note: No article can show you exhaustively how to perform anal fisting safely. If you have never done this and you want to try, do your homework. But you also need to meet people who are already in this scene. Watching others play, trying it out with expert mentoring, and listening to verbal instruction or feedback is still the best way to learn how to do this safely. Besides, if you don't find seasoned fisters, what good is all this book learning going to do you?

Fantasies
and Philosophies

CHAPTER 11

STOP, DROP, AND ROLE!
EROTIC ROLE PLAYING

MOLLENA WILLIAMS

"Let's pretend…" To us as children, these words opened myriad worlds and possibilities. A simple cardboard box was our spaceship, Dad's old sweater was a cape, and we were off into uncharted territory, limited only by our fertile and unhindered imaginations.

For better, or for worse? Imagination and games of make-believe are often shunned as "childlike things" that grown-ups simply do not do. Yet today, over 12 million people around the world eagerly spend hours a day playing *World of Warcraft*, let alone the hundreds of other massive multiplayer online role-playing games.

I am, among many things, an actor and a performer, and I have been practicing my craft professionally since I was about four years old. But even for me, with a lifetime of formal training and experience under my belt, turning up the heat in bed by playing make-believe sex games can sometimes feel awkward, vulnerable, or difficult.

So why is it so tough for so many of us to stretch our imaginations into our sex lives? There are many reasons why people shy away from using fantasy and role playing to enhance and enrich their sex. Some worry about feeling silly. It can be a serious buzzkill if you feel self-conscious and awkward in the midst of a hot-'n-heavy humping! Furthermore, pretending to be someone you are not or creating a fanciful scenario might seem easy, but sustaining it can be daunting; it's pretty much guaranteed that no one wants to risk being a flop in bed!

It is risky, too. What if you work up the nerve to share with your partner(s) that you have a really hot abduction and ravishment fantasy, only to see them recoil in horror, decry your desires as "weird," or worse yet, "sick," and possibly jeopardize the relationship?

And at its heart, it is intimidating. We often become so accustomed to one style, one approach, one dance move that works for us that flipping the script can be scary. What if you mess it up? Forget the lines? Decide halfway through that you just aren't into it and want out?

All these concerns are valid. However, it is important to remember that fantasy and play are things we are *born knowing how to do*. All you have to do to take that first step is to *remember*. Remember the fearlessness, remember being invested in having fun, remember that there is nothing to lose when you throw yourself wholeheartedly into your play.

As someone who identifies as profoundly kinky, I can say that role playing is one of the things that brought me to a more comfortable place about my own twisted sexuality. Though I felt deeply conflicted about being submissive, and it did not sit well with my fiercely feminist heart, I could *pretend* to be submissive—you know, for science. These games allowed me to playfully investigate a newly unearthed part of my psyche and to become more comfortable with it. It felt safer for me to make-believe my way into a new realm. I gradually understood that this was a big part of who I am, and expressing it freely was precisely what feminism was all about. Nowadays, I do not have to pretend. I can just be me.

For many folks, that is as much as they need. The play's the thing! For others, role playing frees them to explore undiscovered countries in their internal landscapes—to plumb the depths of all that their spirit and imagination has to offer!

There are varied approaches to role playing. Finding one that is right for you will give you a comfortable, fun, sexy way to harness your creative energy.

SIMPLE "WHAT IF…?"

You do not have to come up with elaborate costuming, props, scenery, and character analysis to do some very basic role-playing scenarios. Just be yourself. You've been doing it for a while, so that part should be easy! In the "What if…?" game, you imagine a scenario in which you and your partner(s) may fully engage *as yourselves*. Are you perhaps the disgruntled and weary traveler faced with a *very* invasive search at the hands of a presumptuous, lascivious TSA agent? Or perhaps you are the CEO of a Fortune 500 company, you've been caught inappropriately using your expense account funds, and you would do anything—anything at all—to escape being turned over to the authorities by the CFO.

Imagining how *you*, the you that you are now, would react in those situations is a great way to start your explorations into role playing. You can imagine how you would react because we do that all the time. We all are expert "armchair quarterbacks" when it comes to deciding how we would react in someone else's shoes. Whether second-guessing a referee's call or shouting in dismay when the girl in the horror flick foolishly walks into that dark-ass basement, we *always* have a plan of action that's better than the puerile efforts of the people we are observing.

So go for it. Perhaps you have a real-life scenario you would like to recreate. That crossing guard on whom you had a crush, the hot cop who pulled you over. You can even role-play on the phone. The sexy voice answering your call to customer service? Perhaps the conversation strays to more seductive topics than the annual fee on your credit card account, and you find yourself under the spell of an anonymous, velvet-throated stranger. Once you put on your "How do I make this hot?" glasses, opportunities to sex up quotidian scenarios will blossom all around you.

Sharing real-life experiences with your lover can be amazing foreplay. People love to hear stories, and the opportunity to tell a story with real-time skin-on-skin interaction in the mix can be an exotically delicious treat. Or perhaps you have a knack for the written word? Craft an erotic email, or write up a sexy short story about the scenario you are envisioning, offer to send it to your partner or read it to them[1] as a bedtime story, or perhaps leave them a voicemail if you are the shy type. The very act of sharing is a wonderful way to break open your reluctance and get your partner's buy-in. It can help you build trust, which in turn helps you relax into the possibilities and enjoy the ride.

We have all heard the maxim "The brain is the biggest sex organ," and what is going on upstairs certainly has a lot to do with the human arousal cycle. Bring your imagination to play when you are engaging your senses in sex—it's an awesome way to open new realms of possibility for that gray matter to explore.

FLASHBACKS

Besides creating a scenario out of the whole cloth of pure imagination, you can role-play a situation you've previously experienced, or revive a moment from the past. Interestingly, for some people who are emotionally invested in their role-play lives, these scenes may not always be hottest and sexiest. Some people revisit memories of a traumatic or difficult situation through role play to shift the outcome and reclaim their power. If you have faced racism, sexism, or discrimination based on your gender, body type, or socioeconomic status, there is a rich source of role play to be mined here.

You can also cut and paste from your history. It may be wildly insensitive to turn to your lover and say, "Hey, I'm gonna close my eyes and pretend you are this ex-partner of mine who was simply an amazing lover, okay?" Creating a role-play scenario focusing on what made your ex such a delightful sexual

> *Role-playing can free you from the occasional hesitancy many of us feel when asking for exactly what we want.*

partner is far more intriguing. Was there a situation, a place, a time that brings you back? Did you have a particular shirt that your lover removed from you in just a certain way that left you hungry for more? Perhaps an unexpected caress in a surprising place that drove you wild? Share and then dare to go there, because most folks want to learn how to get more pleasure out of their sexual experiences. And who better than you to show your partner how you like to be done?

Role-playing can free you from the occasional hesitancy many of us feel when asking for exactly what we want. And it also permits you to cherry-pick from your sexual history to gather the highlights and craft a scenario that embraces all the heat and fire and passion that you recall from your favorite encounters. Only this time you can skip over the awkward parts and get right to the hot hotness!

YOU'RE SUCH A CHARACTER!

We have plenty of adulation for those performers who can morph chameleon–like into varying personae. It can be truly amazing when a skilled actor seems to blend seamlessly into the character they are portraying, losing themselves in the process. One of the wonderful benefits of role playing is that you can step outside the person you are in your "default" life and become someone entirely different. This type of role playing, "becoming the other," gives you a unique freedom.

If it is in your nature to be aggressive, demanding, and extroverted, try adopting a character who is shy, retiring, and bashful. This gives you room to explore a reality that, while it might not be where you want to live, is a liberating place to visit. And if you tend to be the sort for whom even making a move on someone you find attractive seems a massive impossibility, take on the persona of a consummate seducer—give yourself permission to be the passionate Casanova, Cleopatra, siren, or succubus. Be the irresistible creature of everyone's fantasy. Inhabiting that character can expose a facet of you that you might not even know is there!

Let slip your ideas of gender, race, body type—none of these matter when you use your head to get out of your body. Don't worry about who you think you are right now. Turn your gaze inward, open yourself to the possibility of becoming, even if for just a little while, someone else. If I want to have crazy monkeysex with my partner while pretending I am a captured rōnin Samurai, I am not gonna let it stop me that the body I currently inhabit just so happens to be that of a curvy black woman. A little research, a little creativity, and I can find myself in excruciating Japanese rope bondage being mercilessly interrogated by a ruthless overlord who is bent on sullying my honor with whatever, uh, tools are at their disposal.

DRAWING THE LINE

Your fantasies do not have to be politically correct. They do not have to be socially acceptable. It is not pathological or abnormal to have fantasies that incorporate rape, abduction, sexual abuse, nonconsensual violence, racial bigotry, or any of the behaviors that constitute "man's inhumanity to man." While negotiation with and the consent of all involved parties is vital to a safe, sexy, and fun role-playing romp, the sky is the limit when it comes to doing what you want to do.

At the core of role playing is the truth that we all have within us many, many facets. It can be difficult, especially for those of us raised in a social atmosphere of repression, to let go of the idea that we might be "wrong" or "sick" if we have darker fantasies. The truth of it is, we *all* have our darker fantasies, and those shadowy places can be a rich playground, too. Of course, these fantasies add a layer of complexity when you take on a role or persona with a sinister aspect.

First, it can be troubling to see your own appetite for destruction brought into the light. It can also be surprising to discover how we react when confronted with our demons, or with the monsters that live in those we love and care for. But I do not believe that we ought to shy away from these scary creatures or avoid fearsome fantasies. Fantasies of rape, humiliation, and degradation are not uncommon. But the shame we frequently attach to these desires can hamper us from

> The truth of it is, we all *have our darker fantasies, and those shadowy places can be a rich playground, too.*

exploring them, and therefore knowing ourselves. The core issue is not that what you do is "wrong" or "bad"; it is that you may *feel* wrong or bad because of messages you have received from society or family. When you act out your fantasies, you can leave all that behind.

Many of us are raised to feel shame as sexual beings. But consenting adults who are able to embrace their desires and make them flesh have the unique advantage of moving beyond shame and guilt. We do so in a spirit of liberating and exploring our sexuality. But always keep in mind your limits—your boundaries, the stuff you just cannot or will not do. When negotiating your fantasies with your partners, make clear what is and is not okay. It might be hot to pretend you're the naughty schoolgirl being ravished by a stern teacher, but if you are a survivor of abuse, this type of role play might trigger a flashback to that trauma, bring up a bad memory, or cause a reaction that is not conducive to hot consensual sex. Make sure you talk about your past and get clear on your motives and your desires before engaging in this play.

"I WANNA DO BAD THINGS TO YOU." NEGOTIATE THIS!

Negotiation, limits, and consent are of *critical* importance when exploring role playing. Without them, you increase the risk of missteps that can derail the fun, or worse, create emotional chaos. Even a light, fun scene can be derailed if expectations are not clear and everyone is not on the same page.

When thinking about and planning these scenes, consider

your own and your partner's motivations, desires, likes and dislikes, wants and needs. As I said, the sky's the limit, but you have to decide to go there together. The negotiation process—setting boundaries for what is or is not acceptable, working out the desired scenario, deciding how long the scene will last—can seem a bit of a bore and a big old chore.

> Some folks are wonderful when it comes to improvisation and winging it; others absolutely need to know what is around the bend in order to feel safe.

But consider it foreplay. Try whispering into your lover's ear that you just bought this hot bondage gear and you're wondering how long it might last while you're securely pinned down and at their mercy. Make the negotiation part of the scene. You can get their buy-in to the scenario during the negotiation process, and if it happens in an organic, sexy environment, it won't feel like work at all.

Setting boundaries is important no matter what roles you are considering. Whether you are the passive captive, the aggressive ravisher, or embodying your younger, more innocent self, losing your virginity in the backseat of a '57 Chevy, ya gotta know where the edges of things are. Some folks are wonderful when it comes to improvisation and winging it; others absolutely need to know what is around the bend in order to feel safe. Be clear about your own boundaries, and make sure you are crystal clear about the boundaries of your partner.

Telling each other sexy and explicit stories about your fantasy scenarios can be a great negotiation tool. Many people enjoy hearing a rollicking raunchy tale, and this may well be the key to your own secret garden. While it is scary to be vulnerable in this way, it definitely increases your chances of seeing your fantasy become a reality.

"PSST... WHAT ARE YOU WEARING?" DRESS FOR SUCCESS

While it is true that you can use your imagination, and that's pretty much all you need, it can be exciting to add a layer of verisimilitude to your role playing with costuming, props, and location. Jeans and a T-shirt might work well if you are pretending to be a truck driver waylaid and seduced by a hot hitchhiker, but the Dread Pirate Roberts might not be as believable sweeping his captured prince off his feet in the same garb. As an actor, one of my favorite points in the rehearsal process is when we meet our costumes for the first time. I start to understand something deeper about my character when I feel my body enrobed in what they are wearing. Clothes evoke a whole range of emotions. They can arouse, titillate, confine, release, display, hide, and thrill us in many different ways.

Consider what fabrics excite you. Do silk and satin arouse your skin and your mind? Or does the thick hide of a leather jacket, the smell of it, turn your senses to full-on arousal with every creak? Think about what in you is touched by fabrics, textures, clothing. Think about how you might incorporate a particular item of clothing into your scenario. I'm a pretty kinky chick, and I wear all manner of fetish clothing as a matter of business. But a pair of simple white cotton panties and knee socks can send me into a grinning reverie that'll keep me hot and bothered all day long.

Find something that works for you, be it gingham, burlap, chiffon, or cashmere. Feel the texture, absorb the sensual nature of it, think about why it arouses you, and then consider ways to bring it into your encounter.

Your clothes convey a message, and you can manipulate your outward appearance in order to manifest yourself or your character in many ways. If being in a suit makes you feel strong and confident, could fucking in a suit bring a new level of power and a frisson of desire to that scene? What happens if the person being taken is naked and vulnerable, while their partner is fully dressed? For some women, wearing high-heeled shoes is a daily occurrence and doesn't resonate much. But take a person who feels awkward in the shoes, or is acculturated to feel that wearing such footwear is not appropriate for them due to gender roles, and wearing those high-heeled shoes can become a sexually charged transgressive act. Always had short hair? An inexpensive wig ordered online can put you right into the head space of that sexy silver-screen siren you've envied your whole life.

Dressing up is *fun*. Bringing an awareness of what accoutrements turn you on can add to that fun. Even mundane objects can be imbued with a sexy vibe: I had a very intense sexual encounter that was kicked up a notch when my partner and I dared each other to keep our glasses on during the entire fuck. You will not know how difficult it can be to keep your specs on while pounding the headboard until you've tried it.

Whether you are a full-on Renaissance Faire devotee or

just happen to have an old Halloween costume gathering dust in the closet, you can up the ante by dressing to impress. And dressing to undress.

INCORPORATING THOSE PESKY REAL-LIFE CONCERNS

Make-believe is fantastic and I am all for it. However, we must remember that we aren't really Superman and Wonder Woman. Hot, spontaneous romps in the hay have their appeal, but issues such as safer sex, emotional health, and physical limitations have to be taken into account.

It can seem like a drag or a bit out of character to have to get that condom in play, or to have those gloves ready to go, but incorporating them into your scene is, for many folks, a must. Some people choose to suspend disbelief for just a moment (if you read books or watch movies or TV you do this all the time, so hop to it!), then they get their safer-sex shtick together and carry on. Some scenarios lend themselves to all sorts of play specific to protection. Think of a medical exam where your gynecologist or proctologist gets a little…overenthusiastic with those palpations, for example. Those gloves and dental dams can be an even more arousing addition to the play. I know more than a few people who even become aroused at the sound of a glove being snapped on!

And this level of play can have a wonderful benefit, too: by making your safer-sex routine a part of your play, you grab it back from the realm of the awkward and mundane and put it firmly where it should be—a place where you show yourself and your partners that you want to stay healthy and let the play go on and on.

While these games can be fun, they can also be strenuous on the body. Cut yourself some slack. If you want to play caveman, go ahead, but if you throw your lover over your shoulder and bellow, "Og take Grog back to cave for *bump-bump!*" you might end up with Og on the floor with a herniated disc. Be gentle! Know your body's limits. The character you are playing might be a superhero, but you still have to take into account stuff like gravity, flexibility, and how often you use that gym membership when you're getting it on. Be safe. Don't overdo it while you're doing it.

It's also important to know where you are, emotionally. Role playing can be fun and silly, but it can also touch on some serious emotional issues. When negotiating and engaging in role play, be prepared for the chance that you may unearth complex feelings and the play may quickly feel very real. That's why you have a safeword—don't be afraid to use it. *Don't be afraid to stop!* Stopping because you aren't sure everything's OK is a better option than pushing through a situation that might lead to a difficult aftermath. When in doubt, tap out! There is always another day.

WHAT HAPPENS NOW? AFTERCARE AND REENTRY

So you've just done your epic Tarzan and Jane scene, and maybe Cheetah is a bit worn out. Everyone is lying there in a big quivering pile of sweat-soaked bliss. On your average night it might be enough to do an otter roll in the sheets and a round of Rock/Paper/Scissors to see who gets the wet spot. But if you have just been romping about in the borrowed robes of your hot sexy scenario, a bit more consideration might be in order. Sometimes the role play is foreplay, in which case the sex is a denouement, and may be separate from the scene. Or the sex can be the very center of the scene, vital to the story you and your lover, or lovers, are weaving for each other. Whatever the case, think about what you may need in the aftermath. It's a great way to improve your chances of a safe landing.

Playing can take you to new and exciting places. But afterward? You have to find a way back. Knowing how you tend to react after sex is something you would do well to consider when you are plotting your nefarious role-playing deeds. If one of you tends to fall right asleep and the other turns into Spider-Man and has to be pried off the ceiling after sex, you can run into some issues!

I know my own reaction can vary. Some sex puts me right into "Touch me and die, fool!" mode, while at other times I want to cuddle and snuggle—or jump up and whip up a three-course meal. This unpredictability can be even more challenging when you are coming off channeling a character or unfurling a scenario that was a journey to a very different place.

Stay open and remain compassionate in the time immediately postplay—it's a good way to come back down to earth and to focus on the most important element in the role play: the people involved. Sure, it is hot to pretend. But at the core of the role play are the players. Acknowledging that you had a great time with your play partner(s) helps reinforce the connection you've made with them. And it can help restore their humanity, in case it was compromised by the scene. It can be uncomfortable to feel that you were merely a pawn in another's fantasy—unless of course, your fantasy *is* to be someone's hapless pawn!—so in the reentry phase I like to reconnect, check in, to give reassurance that I am present for them. And I ask the same of them for my well-being.

Think about what you might need in terms of postplay sustenance, and have it handy. After you've bridged the gap between fantasy and reality, it is a great idea to debrief and see how it was for all involved parties. Things might come up for you immediately or take some time to bubble to the surface. Listening and discussing how things went can lay an excellent foundation for the next time you choose to go spelunking in your imagination.

Whatever turns you on, whatever the intent of your fantasy, whatever your desired level of complexity, ultimately this is about you—satisfying your desires and exploring parts of yourself that you might not be able to access every day or any other way. From the tender and mild to the whole-hog buck-wild, your fantasies are as individual as your fingerprints.

Exploring your sexuality by trying out other characters, creatures, or personae is as ancient as humanity and as cutting-edge as technology. Whether it is quickie in an alley or a scenario that takes weeks to plan and nine friends to pull off, adding your most vivid imaginings to your sexual alchemy is a fantastic way to bring your deeper self, or selves, to light. Leave behind your apprehension, step out of your nervousness, and be you, elevated and expanded and limitless.

So, sure, go ahead and order the full Klingon ensemble with prostheses for your head, download the Klingon language tutorials. Or maybe just turn to your lover tonight and say, "Lets pretend you are me, and I am you." And take that leap.

Endnotes

1   I deliberately use the plural pronouns *they*, *them*, and *their* to refer to singular persons of any gender, in place of "he or she," "him or her," "his or her." Although this is nonstandard grammatical usage, the traditional forms reflect a gender binary to which I do not subscribe.

CHAPTER 12

A ROMP ON THE WILD SIDE: EROTIC HUMAN ANIMAL ROLE PLAYING

LEE HARRINGTON

THE CALL OF THE WILD

The call of being something other than human appeals to many of us. As kids, we pretended to be wolves hunting in the woods, trotted around being pretty ponies, or curled up on the floor and had fun as a spoiled house cat. That desire is still present for many of us, and in the world of kinky and adventurous sex you too can be something other than human—or have a human animal all your own.

Each person is called to animal role playing for their own reasons. Perhaps you like having fun and being silly, or you're looking for an outlet for letting go of stress. How many of us have tough days at the office and just would like to be "something else" for a while? After all, puppies don't think about paying taxes, and being a dragon means not worrying about whether the dishes need to be done.

All forms of role playing let us step out of being ourselves for a while. We try on a different role, a different mask, a different character. We transform into plundering pirates, wicked dominatrices, and naughty schoolgirls.

> *When we take away our human masks to become more animalistic, sometimes core parts of our identity come to the forefront.*

The same is true for human animal role playing. When we get to be an animal for a period of time, we set aside our day-to-day concerns and just have fun with the interactions.

For some, animal role playing is a chance to connect with a partner. By becoming a puppy, we are reliant upon our partner to care for us and our needs, and in doing so we might be able to build trust with our partners in ways we never did before. As the owner or handler of a human animal, we can learn to see our partner in a new light—as playful, loving, feisty, bratty, proud, delicate, service-minded, or strong.

When we take away our human masks to become more animalistic, sometimes core parts of our identity come to the forefront in ways that we were unintentionally hiding from the world at large. When I was in Melbourne, Australia, I was invited to attend a human puppy romp, a party night at a fetish club called Chains. I showed up as "Gunner," my Rottweiler persona. About eight human puppies were there with their handlers, and about 60 other people. I wandered around sniffing crotches and having fun playing with the other puppies, until I noticed a problem. A man had brought his girlfriend to the event as a human pony, and the other dogs were barking at her. She was scared.

I rushed away from the person I was flirting with, still on all fours. I was barking at full volume, a loud angry bark, as I got between the pony girl and the human puppies. Yipping and snapping, they were confused at me—why wasn't I joining the fun and scaring the pony? In that moment I realized that I held a core value that the fun of others is never worth the true suffering of another. It was through my own animal role playing that I realized how deeply I felt about my own convictions.

Desire and Dress

Sexiness and an outright erotic turn-on can call many to animal role playing. I have met sensual snakes who liked to taste every inch of their lovers' flesh before squeezing down tight, and well-hung pony boys ready to be used as the studs they are. Animal role playing is about sexually consenting adults choosing to dress up or play pretend as if they were animals. It should not be confused with bestiality, in which humans are erotically involved with actual animals. Those who are turned on by animal role playing have sex with their human partners, who happen to be animal characters, and they may or may not be using the role playing to play with a specific taboo.

Sometimes it is all about the wardrobe. That inexpensive pair of kitty-cat ears you wore at Halloween a few years ago with the slinky matching outfit? You were doing animal role playing! Some people go all-out with wardrobe or fetish wear, investing in hoof-shaped boots, mitts to take away the use of their hands, makeup that expresses their primal self, or hoods shaped like the face of their animal persona or character. There are even butt plugs available on the market nowadays that look like pony tails, puppy tails, and even curly pigtails in pink.

Wardrobe isn't just for the animals either. How many of us have lusted after the smart-looking woman in an English riding costume, or the bad-boy dog-fighting trainer? Whether dressing up in jodhpurs and boots or a sexy jogging outfit, we as the human counterparts to our animal characters can have fun with costuming as well.

For those more attracted to complex costumes, there is an entire community known as *Furries* or Furry Fandom. Role-playing anthropomorphic animals (such as walking, talking lions) rather than "realistic" animals, the Furry community is a blend of science-fiction fandom, cosplay (Japanese costume/character-based role playing) and costume aficionados, and erotic role players. Not all Furries see themselves as being into erotic animal role playing—so don't assume that just because someone plays dress-up they want to "yif" with you (engage sexually while in character or role as Furries). Some Furries wear complete mascot costumes, while others are happy in just ears and a tail—or they may consider their animal identity always in place, even when not in costume.

Body, Mind, and Spirit

Perhaps you are drawn to animal role playing because it is a chance to actively engage with your physical body. Many of us wander around partially disconnected from our bodily experience. We ignore that our back hurts sitting at our office desk, or tune out the noises of living in big cities. By becoming an animal, we have a chance to be fully present in our bodies; we might be petted or brushed down, engaging with our skin through sensation play. Perhaps it is a chance to activate our muscles by challenging our body, for example, in role as a strong horse, pulling a cart that our partner is sitting in. Our olfactory sense might come to the forefront when we take the time to actually smell and taste the world around us—licking our partner's body and smelling them inch by inch.

Some individuals are drawn to animal role play through their spirituality. Whether working with totems, feeling connected to animal spirits, or being drawn to the energy of the werewolf, these individuals feel an energetic connection to the animal in question. They may or may not perceive themselves as *Therian*—having the energetic body of an animal that does not match their physical form as a human. For animal role players rooted in spirituality, this practice is profound and deeply meaningful. In fact, many role players have had moments of epiphany or other spiritual insights through their opportunity to see the world from a different perspective.

CHOOSE YOUR ANIMAL

Whatever our reason for engaging in animal role playing, there are many ways to tailor it to your desires. We can choose the species we play, its personality, what characters we interact with, and of course what kinds of activities we get up to (and the characters we interact with in those activities). Just choose one item from each of the three categories below—species, personality, and interactions—and you're ready to go!

Species

Human animals come in species great and small. People who are drawn to horses and ponies engage in *pony play*. Pony players are often drawn to the equine features of strength, elegance, beauty, grace, power, poise, and confidence. Some want to be show ponies, prancing for spectators and being fed sugar cubes for their coordinated routines. Perhaps the chance to be a sweaty workhorse calls more to you—pulling your partner in a cart up a hill and being washed down by their firm hands afterward. Other pony and horse archetypes include the feisty filly, stud stallion, old nag ready for the glue factory, wild Palomino, focused workhorse, skittish pony, queen of the parade, and the foal on new legs.

The next most common species for animal play is canine (dogs, puppies, and wolves). *Puppy players* find commonality with and inspiration from the canine traits of camaraderie, playfulness, devotion, and bravery. Others enjoy puppy play because it gives them the chance to be a horny dog in heat, someone's best friend, or the chance to be bouncy and playful as a young puppy. Human puppies are given a fantastic view of the world, seeing everyone at crotch level. Some examples of puppy play archetypes are the yappy Toy Poodle, sled dog, alpha wolf, prized Chihuahua, kennel bitch, loving Labrador, lonely Basset Hound, Boxer in heat, and Rottweiler guard dog.

Felines are another often-desired animal species for role players. *Kitty play* might involve role playing as a cat or a kitten, or even wild feline species such as lions, leopards, or tigers. Some are drawn to the loving feline traits of being cuddly, playful, sweet, or sensual, while others are called by the standoffish, aloof, and proper demeanor of some cats. Cats, after all, often exhibit an extreme dichotomy of traits, and this appeals to a number of role-playing possibilities. Kitty play archetypes include the pretty kitty, lost kitten, cranky house tabby, troublemaking alley cat, cowardly lion, and wild bobcat.

Though pony play, puppy play, and kitty play get the most air time in the world of animal role playing, there are many other species to choose from. Farm animals appear often in animal role play pornography, where girls are depicted as cows being milked and gay piggy boys roll around wallowing in the mud. Fans of erotic humiliation might be drawn to worm and bug roles, where a dominant partner can "squish" their partner underfoot or treat them for the length of the scene as worthless and small.

Birds of all shapes are a fantastic inspiration for role playing: think of trained parrots, wild pigeons, elegant swans, or precocious penguins. In the public kinky sex community I've played with a human ferret who traveled with its own jingly toys, and it would not be surprising to meet a human rat or mouse. How many of us have enjoyed the aesthetics of scantily clad bunny girls? If you are not drawn to the simple, consider becoming something more exotic—a zebra, monkey, dolphin, snake, or hippopotamus. Even the occasional dinosaur, dragon, or sphinx has been known to make an appearance in bedroom fantasy adventures.

Personality

Once we have an idea of the kind of species we would enjoy being, we can explore our pet personality. Would you rather have your animal persona be close to your daily demeanor or something radically different? For example, if you are easy-going in your day-to-day life, you might enjoy an opposite role, like a defensive Doberman; maybe you want to be more like your average self but in dog form, like a happy-go-lucky Golden Retriever.

Neither is better or worse, but it is important to consider what traits call to you today. You can choose a different personality next time. Do you want your pet personality to be lazy? Feisty and bratty? Do you want to use your pet self as a chance to explore submission or service? Perhaps your darker desires come to the surface and you want a safe framework to explore being an abused pony (literally kicked when they are down), or a feral wolf on the hunt for blood.

If unsure in which direction to take your character's personality, consider some animal names. Are you Lady? Piglet? Lancelot? Beast? Pinky? Boxer? Lord Eduardo, King of the Goats? Names hold a lot of power. Being called by our pet name gets us out of our day-to-day space and into our role. They also tell us a lot about the personality of the pet and how to interact with them. An ironic combination of species and name can also be hilarious, affecting how we treat both the pet and their handler. Most of us would react differently to a Chihuahua named Pinky than we would to a Pit Bull named Pinky.

INTERACTIONS

Reason for play, species, and personality in hand—now what? Now we get to decide what characters we interact with. Will you be a pet on your own, playing with toys or eating from a bowl? Will a human puppy play with another human puppy, or a group of human puppies, at a kinky sex conference? Perhaps your inner house cat and your partner's puppy will interact with one another.

Others will want to have their animal self interact with a human character. There is a lot of enjoyment to be had by being one of these humans. Do you want to be a pet "owner," having pride in your pet, investing in or showing off a top-valued racehorse, or bonding with what is yours? For human pet owners, there is an intimacy of connection that can arise as pet and owner grow into their roles together.

Sometimes a pet "trainer" actually spends more time with a pet than its owner does. Trainers have the capacity to create a regimen, formality, and structure with a human animal as they train it how to behave. You might enjoy being a trainer (or playing with one) if you enjoy dominance and submission, or if the notion of positive or negative reinforcement gets your juices flowing. By pushing or cajoling the creature, trainers help push their animal into being the best animal they can be.

Sometimes a pet just needs to connect with a handler, someone who is a fan of pets and likes interacting with them without being invested as a trainer or owner. These are folks who have fun petting the kitty, playing tug-of-war with the puppy, or riding around on the pony's back. Being a handler can be a great chance to let go of stress, fulfill our need for a nonhuman pet by having a human one step in, or explore bestiality fantasies.

ACTIVITIES

Many animal role players get flustered about what to do as human animals and their handlers. It's okay. When you see porn featuring thousand-dollar pony harnesses, hoof boots, and a full farm to be run around in, it can feel as if you'll never go there without the financial investment. This is not true.

One of the simplest ways to encourage your transformation into an animal role is by changing your physicality into that of your animal of choice. Yes, those hoof boots might make you stand taller and walk upright, but so can a pair of high heels, or just standing taller and prouder. Consider petting your pony's back to remind her of her posture, or physically straighten her out. Head high, proud! Even if he is a four-legged pony (someone who goes around on hands and knees, sometimes offering ponyback rides for those their frame can safely hold), help your pet keep good posture and his head high. Thus you can create physicality with no cost at all.

Physicality can be encouraged in two-legged pony play (walking on human legs) by binding the arms back with something as simple as a pair of cuffs. For cats and dogs, encourage them to ball their hands in mitts, get a pair of gardening or sports knee pads to let them crawl around for longer on all fours, or find some sort of tail that can move as they crawl or walk about. For worms, what about binding the arms at their sides? What will help them be the pet they want to be?

Once you are physically moving like an animal, consider the types of activities your animal enjoys. Horses can be trotted around a room, led on a lead for formal dressage training, or hooked up to a cart for pulling. They might be put on display and examined at a human animal "show," set up to be "studded," or brushed down after a sweaty afternoon of activity (a great way to explore unusual sensations). Puppies can also be brushed, but what about feeding them a dish of chili out of a bowl on the floor—it looks a lot like dog food. Cats might be petted by their favorite little girl, or get taken to the vet. This allows for animal role play to be combined with age play (where grown adults pretend to be younger) or medical play (where a fetish for medical tools and wardrobe is engaged).

> *Come to it with a sense of humor and a willingness to see what evolves, instead of having a picture of the outcome in mind the very first time.*

Start out small. Try exercises like crawling on the ground, eating without your hands, or chasing a laser beam around a room. What does it feel like to curl up under your lover's legs and let her pet you for a while? Come to it with a sense of humor and a willingness to see what evolves, instead of having a picture of the outcome in mind the very first time.

If you find that the characters everyone plays are enjoyable, consider moving up to more complex wardrobe, props, or activities. A first-time scene is not the best time to invest in the milking equipment and full Swedish country girl costume—save that for after you know everyone is actually into it. Why spend the money, time, or energy on it if you don't even know whether you and your partner will enjoy animal role playing?

Find inspiration in the animals you mimic. What types of play do they engage in at home in their native environments? How do they notify their humans when they are hungry or need to answer the call of nature? What kinds of noises do they make and how do they move? These are all great places to draw ideas for role playing.

CARE AND FEEDING

When we engage in human animal role playing, the partner who becomes the pet is offering himself, his love, and his trust as a gift. With that level of trust, it is important that you, as the handler of a human pet, keep up your side of the bargain and care for him while you are in role.

Does this mean that handlers need to provide for all the needs of their play partners? No. Before everyone gets into character, it is best to decide who is responsible for bringing what items, props, beverages etc. to the scene. Many pets have a preferred head harness, favorite chew toy, or precious fluffy bunny tail. Use them! They are already attached to those items and it will allow them more chances to be fully in role. Make sure someone remembers food, water, safer-sex supplies, explicitly erotic toys, and anything else that might come in handy during the scene.

During play, also keep in mind what systems of communication you will use. In many forms of kinky sex play, people use a safeword to let others know when they need to check in or stop the scene, but many human animal role players prefer not to use human speech. If you are playing with someone who wants to be able to communicate a safeword or needs to check in while staying in role, consider alternate systems, such as picking up a toy you otherwise would not use or rhythmically stomping a paw or hoof.

Some pets drop so deeply into their role that they can only understand their trainer's body language and tone once they are fully transformed into their animal self. These human animals may not be able to deliver safewords or warn you that they are tired of using human words—so find out what their language is. When they are tired, do they yawn or try to lie down? When they are hurt, do they buck up and try to get away? This could be mistaken for obstinacy—find out why your pet mews or screams.

Ethics

The issue of ethics also comes up when we are playing with those who drop so deeply into role that they no longer can communicate with us in human language. Just as BDSM has *subspace*, where a bottom goes so deeply into submission that it may be a challenge for them to communicate, this can happen with some animal role players. If this happens to your partner, consider whether you should honor what you agreed to before they went into character or listen to what the animal before you is trying to tell you.

Things can sometimes go wrong. Once, shooting with Playboy television, I was being ridden by starlet Kira Reed while I was a four-legged pony. I had been a pony for some time that day, and my head space had slipped into being that of a horse—I had forgotten how to speak. This would not have been an issue, except that Kira was wearing spurs—she kicked my thighs and I bucked. She thought I was being playful, and so did everyone else on the shoot. She kicked me again, and I bucked again. This went on for some time, my horse self trying to throw her, and Kira digging in deeper. Finally someone saw that I was bleeding from the spurs.

She was mortified. I was slowly brought back to being a human by taking my tack and costume off, bringing me back layer by layer to my human skin. She and I talked about what happened, and we were all fine, but it taught me that if you plan to do anything really physically tough (a horse-breaking scene or a greased pig catch, say), consider working out nonverbal cues as a form of safeword. If the animal comes to a dead stop, for example, it's a good sign that something is wrong. If they are not fully in animal head space and can talk, try using a partial language system. Many folks use stomping or barking to indicate yes and no—one bark, yes, two barks, no. Other options involve pet versions of head shakes—up and down for yes, side to side for no. Perhaps you will develop a system where someone needing to go to the bathroom will paw at the bathroom door.

Fully character or animal-invested individuals might be fine with playing beyond what you would do with an actual animal, but are you? If you are the handler, trainer, or pet owner, consider what your limits are for playing with individuals who have "become" animals. Perhaps you were delighted to have your sexy kittygirl lick you for hours on end, but if she no longer seems to understand English and is acting like an actual cat, how do you feel about engaging with her sexually? Do you feel it crosses the line into a bestiality fantasy, or is it just good clean fun? It is important to observe these limits during a scene, and discuss your behavior with your partner when they are fully human again.

Training and Correction

But what happens if your pet does something inappropriate? If they are acting a way because it is in alignment with their persona, look at how you might react to an actual animal that had behaved that way. Is it squirt bottle time for the unruly cat, or a swat on the ass with a rolled up newspaper for the naughty puppy? If your pet does something silly—laugh! If he can't open up the plastic bag because he's a kitten in mitts (or has socks taped over his hands), help the poor kitty out. Say, "Poor kitty, let me get that for you." If she's a happy and jumpy puppy and you are trying to focus on a task, chide her like the bad dog she is.

But if your lover or play partner actually does something that upsets you, pause or stop the role playing. Do not try to work out your anger and frustration by using the scene as an excuse to literally kick your human dog. This applies to the animal role player as well. If you and your partner are having a challenge in your life together, don't just pee on the rug to get even. Discuss real issues in a human-to-human dialogue.

Once we have explored the fun and the silliness, the sexiness and the sensuality, the fierceness and more of our characters, some of us may be done. There is nothing wrong with trying out a character once, having fun, and moving on. Others want to come back to their personas again and again, setting regular kitty play date nights or creating a cue to indicate when they are in kitty character, such as putting on a collar.

Remember, this is your scene, your play, your desires. Make human animal role play the best for everyone involved. Let it feel silly, let it feel profoundly intimate and connecting—it's all okay. And if your play has just gone crazy, be willing to do what good pet owners have always done since time immemorial: curse, swear, laugh, spit, cuddle up with your pet, and be in the moment. Tomorrow, maybe you'll switch roles and be Lord Eduardo, King of the Goats.

CHAPTER 13

FORTEFEMME: THE ART AND PHILOSOPHY OF FEMININE DOMINANCE

MIDORI

Do you want to explore your dominant female side? Want to be that take-charge, fierce woman of danger and mystery, who gets what she wants while putting her partners through their paces? Do you want to feel confident in your sensual power, but are uncertain where to start? Or maybe you're having urges of erotic power but are turned off by the tacky clichés of bad bitches? Perhaps your lover has requested you to take control and you find yourself wrestling with confusion and conflict. You're not alone in any of this.

A word about terminology here: In this chapter I use the term *femme* often. I prefer not to define it too narrowly, but rather let it elicit your subjective impression of what is feminine or female. It applies to your inner experience of the feminine, beyond gender and orientation. We all harbor feminine, masculine, and androgyne aspects in ourselves. Here I am addressing the individual expression of the feminine in the state of play and pleasure.

Media and SM fiction would make it seem that the archetypal leather-clad dominant woman springs fully formed from the dark recesses of society, ready to scream like a banshee with whip in hand. The truth is that the real sexually dominant woman walks among us. She's at your workplace. She's on the commute with you. She's strolling past you with a latte in hand. To understand the dominant woman, or to become her, step away from the common kinky expectations and consider who she really is. Strip away the corny SM stereotype, and what you have is a femme in possession of power, sensuality, and most importantly, herself. I'm certain you've met her.

There are the classic icons of sexy dominant women: Dietrich, Cleopatra, Mata Hari, Scheherazade, Lady Murasaki, and Madame Du Barry. There are pop icons of femme power, such as Catwoman, Madonna, Wonder Woman, Lara Croft, and the like. But don't forget the power femme in the everyday woman. She gracefully faces the obstacles and challenges of life with humor and determination, and creates her own success and destiny. That's most certainly a woman of potency and substance. Consider all the challenges you've faced and the confidence you've gained from them. There is a power femme within you, waiting to be unleashed in the bedroom.

The heart of feminine potency and feminine dominance is simple, but far from easy or formulaic. It's confidence. No step-by-step instructional on female domination can teach the confidence that leads to the uniquely sexy allure of the femme. No technical classes on flogging, bondage, or kink skills can create the powerful femme. No collection of leather, corsetry, latex, shoes, or other fetish accessories will make a woman sexually self-actualized. The essence of femme allure is simple, but it is certainly not easy to come by.

HOW TO FIND YOUR POWER SOURCE: THE ARCHETYPE

One of the most effective ways to begin identifying your power femme within is the Archetype Exercise. It'll take a while to do this, so take your time. You will need a piece of paper and a pen.

Consider this question: Who personifies the alluring powerful femme for me?

The question is trickier than it looks. Don't just start writing down names; think carefully about your life, about which women have influenced you with their charisma, their confidence, their sensuality. The answers may be different than you expect. Although the names you write down will be those of other women, this exercise is all about you.

Give answers in as many of the following categories as you can:

Myth and religion
Folktales
History

Politics
Popular culture
TV/movie characters
Family history
Literary characters
Media personalities
Comics/manga/games
Professions
People in your past and present

What names do you come up with? For me, women such as Catherine Deneuve, Mae West, Catwoman, Cleopatra, Amaterasu Omikami (the Japanese sun goddess), Brunnhilde, and my grandmother come to mind. These are but a few in a long list of women I admire for their allure as power femme icons.

Now write those names in a column on the left side of the paper. Write as many as you can think of—the more, the better! You can do it in one sitting, or put down the list and go back to it from time to time. You may also want to bounce the question around with your partner or friends. Other icons for me are the Oiran (the highest-ranking courtesans of Japan), RuPaul, Emma Peel, prison wardens, Lauren Bacall, Borg Queen, or Drill Sergeant Rainey from my own basic training days.

ARCHETYPE EXERCISE WORKSHEET

Name of your powerful femme icon	Their powerful femme attributes (List both the light and the dark aspects)

Once you feel that you've done a pretty thorough job of listing your icons of powerful femininity, focus on each one individually and write down what makes her a power femme for you. You can use words, phrases, or thought fragments. Just brainstorm and let the words flow—don't worry about whether the attributes you're noting are historically accurate. Write down your impressions of these women and what you feel makes them iconically femme and powerful. It's purely subjective.

Take Catherine Deneuve, for example. I can say with confidence that she has a great sense of style. I cannot say with any certainty, however, that she feels vulnerable or that she understands her vulnerability to be part of her power. But I believe Deneuve does just that as an actress, so I would write that down. Some of the traits may not seem complimentary or flattering. Amaterasu Omikami was said to be fickle; Dietrich may have been selfish. Remember that the femme is not always about sweetness and light, or sugar and spice and everything nice. Sometimes the darker qualities of these femmes are exactly what make them so alluring—it is what makes them femmes fatales. Light cannot exist without shadow. Make sure to list the dark attributes as well as the light ones. Do this for all the names you've listed.

You will now have two columns on a piece of paper: your icon names on the left and their attributes on the right. Now put the list aside and go do something fun. Maybe you suddenly feel a need to find a lipstick in the most perfect shade of red. Good. Go and do something that pleases you. With a refreshed mind, revisit the list. Fold the paper so you can only see the attributes column on the right.

This right column is the index of your inner power femme attributes. Are you surprised? What words reappear? What theme is constant? What traits are you uneasy or uncomfortable with? It's difficult to see our own powerful qualities—we look at others and project upon them what we value as femininity and power. They are our mirrors; they do what we wish we could. Sometimes our admiration of these women feels like a guilty pleasure. Why else would the great villainesses be so attractive? Unfortunately, even in the most progressive Western cultures, women are often discouraged from being self-congratulatory. Many women never fully develop their own image of power or honestly acknowledge their own strengths. It's safer and more comfortable to admire the power in others than to recognize and cherish it within us. A residual effect of having been historically the "second sex" is the inability to see the strength within.

Your personal power femme icons are mirrors of your own potential. Recognize this and it will help you reevaluate your concept of feminine power. How does it feel that these iconic women are part of you? What do you value in your own power, the light as well as the dark? To put it another way, if you were your power femme icon, what would give you great pleasure? What would you do? What would you have someone do for you?

When It Doesn't Feel Right
Do you feel blocked about going full tilt using your power and enjoying your dominance? Maybe you're suffering from mismatched expectations. Do you feel put upon by your

partner's demands? Do elements of your power femme attributes conflict with your partner's fantasy? Where desires and expectations conflict, discontent arises. Let's say that your lover thinks a sexually dominant woman should dress, act, talk, and play a certain way. You act on that and it feels odd and awkward. Why? It's because your traits and desires are in conflict with your lover's vision of your part in their fantasy. Drop the expectations and engage in sweet selfishness in the bedroom! This is the arena for asking for what you want and what would please you. If a sexually dominant woman can't be true to her desires, then she's nothing but a puppet acting her way to certain dissatisfaction and burnout.

Your attribute lists should be pretty long. Would you manifest all of these personae or aspects of your power at any given point during play? No. But it would serve you well to find which of these traits best describe you for that night's play. Do you feel demanding, neutering, coy, bitchy, precise, vulnerable, or delicate? Let the elements that ring truest to you in that moment rule your dominant femme space. Call them your moods or appetites, if you wish. You'll be conducting yourself in a manner that is true to your core, not merely play-acting someone else's idea of a sexually dominant woman.

Return to your worksheet and take a look at the left column of power femme icon names. Many of the names that you listed are potential sources of roles for you and your partner to play. If Cleopatra made your list, consider the role of the imperious ancient queen. This gives you plenty of opportunity for dress-up. Dressing up as characters other than your everyday self may feel a bit silly at first, but it's all in the name of fun and pleasure. Read Chapter 11, Stop, Drop, and Role! Erotic Role Playing, and incorporate those skills into your dominant appetites and attributes. Dressing up for SM role-play games can free you from your accustomed good manners and limitations. Maybe you would never order your partner around, but the Queen of the Nile certainly would!

Are you worried that your dominant femme traits in the bedroom might take over your everyday life in negative ways? The act of putting on and taking off role-play costumes provides a clear demarcation of when imperious behavior is appropriate and when it ends. It also gives your partner a clear delineation of when a certain type of relationship starts and ends. It's a healthy way to create boundaries and keep playtime special and distinct.

WHAT REALLY TURNS ON A SUBMISSIVE PARTNER

Here's a dirty little truth: what deeply arouses your partner isn't the long list of activities they listed in their negotiations. There's no doubt that those activities are important and enjoyable; however, it's your presence and delivery that makes or breaks the experience. It's about attitude! If the submissive senses that your heart isn't in it and you're just faking it as you deliver the spankings or other ministrations, it kills the thrill. It's 10 times worse than faking orgasms—which is pretty criminal in itself. The submissive may go along with it just to have an "itch" scratched, while you perform to their expectations—creating a vicious cycle of destructive noncommunication. This can only end in ugly resentments.

In the same way that you now have your personal list of power femme attributes and personae that are authentic to you, every submissive has their list of Dream Domme attributes. Most bottoms and submissives haven't thought about this, as standard SM negotiations tend to focus exclusively on activities at the cost of intention, mood, and emotional needs. Find out what dominant demeanor makes them weak in the knees. If that matches your styles of dominance, you have the golden key to inspiring deep submission and unparalleled joy in them. Now add technically delightful play and you've just created magic for them.

To find out what dominant style your partner is keyed in to, put them through a stealthy version of the Archetype Exercise. You could hand them the form, but since that wouldn't be sexy or fun for many people, disguise it as an ordinary conversation. Perhaps after a movie with a particularly strong female character, or sharing a book with power femme leads, tease out a conversation about who they believe embodies powerful femininity. Ask what makes these women so fantastic. Keep the conversation going, perhaps over several different occasions, and the pattern will emerge clearly. Did they mention words and phrases similar to your own power femme attribute list? If so, you're set for success!

Some of your partner's favorite power femme attributes may not match yours. Don't force them to match—don't try to act like something you're not. For example, you'll never find "ice queen" on my list—I'm just too goofy for that. If I attempted to be the Ice Queen domme, even my best rope bondage scene would feel stiff, staged, and boring. So what to do? I would find another key phrase or attribute that the submissive mentioned that is more my style. Maybe it was "clever," "cruel," "creative," or "controlling." Now, those I can do. They're in my light and dark lists.

Don't hesitate about trying on a new style. If it feels good, keep it and add it to your style list. If it doesn't fit right, drop it from your list and move on. Whatever you do should please you.

THE GOOD DOMINANT

What makes for a dominant of quality? In the flood of information circulating in publications and media and on the net, sometimes the young power femme may feel a bit overwhelmed. It's easy to lose sight of the basics in a frenzy of information gathering.

From the Core

Effective dominance comes from the core of the person. This is why it's essential to know your archetypes and attributes. No amount of fetish wear can make a dominant out of a woman who hasn't

> *No amount of fetish wear can make a dominant out of a woman who hasn't worked on her power and grace within.*

worked on her power and grace within. Having a collection of great toys won't make you a great domme either—it just means that you know where to shop. The same goes for skills. Knowing a lot of techniques does not alone make you a great domme. It'll make you a skilled top, but that's different from being a dominant. You might be a good service top, a lovely submissive sadist, or a fine egalitarian sadist, but these are all different—though no less valid—than being a dominant.

Conversely, you can be dressed in nothing more than ordinary daily clothing, using no equipment and displaying no particular flashy techniques, and still demonstrate deep and powerful dominance.

Know the Domain of Your Influence

A fine domme understands when dominant behavior is appropriate. She knows when to go into domme mode and when to turn it off. She knows that she is not in a Dominant/submissive relationship with the entire world and that the tone and attitude of dominance wielded upon unconsenting people will only earn her their contempt and disrespect. Only misguided, insecure bullies display such behavior. She doesn't let the dominant energy bleed into an egalitarian relationship once a hot scene has ended. If she is in a Dominant/submissive or Master/slave relationship, she understands that her dominance may be expressed differently even within that relationship. What she does in the bedroom or dungeon with her submissives would be quite different from what she would do at the submissive's workplace.

Confidence Is the Root of Power

Never forget that the ultimate aphrodisiac for the sub is the dominant's genuine self-confidence. Sometimes it may come off as cockiness, but the difference between the cocky and the self-confident is the source of validation. The cocky dominant needs to see her greatness reflected in the eyes of others, while

> *The art of the domme is in using her persuasive powers to bring out a desire previously unaroused in the submissive.*

the confident dominant knows what her powers are and accepts them. She has taken inventory of and is comfortable with her own talents, skills, assets, and strengths. She is confident enough to see her own flaws clearly.

If a dominant cracks a whip in the woods and there are no submissives to hear it, is she still a domme? Absolutely! A dominant is not defined by the other—in this case, the presence of a submissive. She is defined by a sense of self and comfort in her own identity as an erotically dominant woman. She knows that the need to define herself by the others around her is a sign of false confidence. Every dominant will find herself single from time to time, whether by circumstance or by choice. Her relationship status does not change who she is fundamentally.

Seduce—Don't Force

The ultimate power is that of persuasion. To get the submissive or bottom to want to do for you what you command of them—that's dominance. Any fool with a scary weapon can force another to do things against his or her will. That's the power of the brutish, the power of fearful people and those lacking in self-confidence. The art of the domme is in using her persuasive powers to bring out a desire previously unaroused in the submissive.

As one of my favorite teachers and authors, Joseph Bean, loves to say: "The number one job of the dominant is to continually seduce consent from the bottom."

Humility Begets Respect

The deep intimacy and connection that genuine Dominance/submission creates verges on magic. There is a moment during the most amazing scenes when the rest of the world melts away, leaving a universe of two, the domme and the sub. In a universe of two, the domme is divine, for that brief moment and in that time-warped space. To accept this, she must be humble. She must know that she is but a mortal woman at all other times.

Such humility has the amazing effect of creating a calm aura around the domme, giving her an air of grace and elegance that is deeply alluring. Her sincere humility and grace earns the domme quiet respect from those around her, and most certainly the respect of her submissive.

Without respect, there is no leadership. Without leadership, there is no dominance, only boorishness.

To Receive Submission, Give Respect and Gratitude

Even the cool and aloof have their ways of showing respect and thanks. A femme domme respects the humanity of the submissive even after the most intense objectification scene. She is thankful for the act of submission given, even when it may appear externally as if it were wrenched from the submissive. She knows that, in the end, it is the submissive who actively chooses surrender. She knows how difficult true surrender is and is in awe of that. She knows that it takes the truly strong and self-aware to fully submit and she shows gratitude for that appropriately.

She knows that the limits and emotional vulnerabilities of

others must be respected. This includes respecting the limits of nonparticipating parties who may prefer not to have to deal with a wantonly splattered dominant attitude. It includes respecting the limits placed by the submissive, for this consideration allows the submissive to feel truly safe with her. Such a sense of safety often leads to deeper surrender. As a dear friend of mine, David V., says: "Always be respectful in spirit, even if the scene is not."

Be True to Your Desires, Your Limits, Your Flaws, and Your Errors

A dominant of quality knows clearly what she enjoys in kink play. If she doesn't, she'll simply be pushed by other people's desires and projected expectations. Like a leaf floating in the current of a fast river, she will be haunted by a vague sense of helplessness and lack of control. What's a dominant if she doesn't have control over her own pleasure? Always know your limits and displeasures just as well as your thrills. The art of the polished domme is in setting boundaries gracefully in such a way that that the submissive delights in this firmness.

She also knows where her flaws and weaknesses are and accepts them. She is strong enough to know that covering up with bravado and pretending her flaws don't exist is a pathetic game played by insecure dominants. She also knows where her technical limitations are and knows how to work around them to avoid undue risk. She knows when to seek more learning to increase her skills, and does so without making each step of dominance education a battle of egos. When she makes an error, which she knows will happen from time to time, she sees the error she has made and acknowledges it. Then she does what needs to be done to correct the situation and moves on. She neither ignores the error nor overreacts to it.

Decisiveness Is Enthralling

The dominant of quality understands the power of decisiveness. Each action is committed with mindfulness, whether arrived at by conscious thought and decision or by instinct. The person who openly waffles in the act appears to have no control. It is fine to wonder about other choices and consider them in one's mind. It is also fine to seek counsel and advice. Do that with decisiveness as well.

The realistic dominant knows that with decisiveness comes the potential for less than optimal outcomes. She strives to be aware of consequences. She takes responsibility for her actions and, once again with decisiveness, grace, and compassion, handles those consequences.

A FEW PRACTICAL TIPS FOR A SCENE

Here are a few basic tips to help you begin creating fulfilling scenes with your partner:

Once you've negotiated a scene with your partner (see Chapter 1 for negotiation tips), put your satisfaction first. Focus on the activities on their wish list that will give you certain pleasure.

Focus on enjoying one or two simple activities thoroughly, even if your partner's wish list is as long as your arm. It's better to do a few things well than many things poorly. Leaving them wanting more is a very desirable thing.

The blindfold is your friend. Blindfolded, every touch and action you create is a thrilling mysterious pleasure for your partner. Blindfolded, your lover will not see you fumbling, expressing bafflement, or removing your high heels.

Whenever you feel uncertain, take a slow breath and ask yourself, What would please me right now? Then follow through with what would please you.

Engage power femme posture! Stand up straight, hold your head high, roll your shoulders back, lift your chest, and pull your navel toward your uterus. Try this in scene and out of scene, and feel how it affects your sense of confidence.

To reduce the possibility of scene failure, begin and end the scene with activities that both of you enjoy, and try new activities in the middle. If a new activity doesn't work for either of you, at least you'll wrap up with pleasure, familiarity, and confidence.

Dominant femmes deserve after-scene care. What would you like that to be? Ask for it before the scene and insist upon it after the scene.

Learn and practice whenever the opportunity presents itself. Take as many classes and educational events as you can. Try classes on topics new, exotic, scary, or mysterious to you. Workshops are great places to explore these subjects safely while giving you space to decide whether you like it.

Have fun! Whether your style is sweet and nurturing or fierce and demanding, or anything in between, remember that this is always about pleasure.

Enjoy your journey and savor your pleasures.

CHAPTER 14

SUBMISSIVE: A PERSONAL MANIFESTO

MADISON YOUNG

I'm a mom. I'm a submissive. I'm a feminist. I struggle to write these words, finding myself in the greatest power play dynamic of my life with a three-month-old infant who lies sleeping in my lap while I hunch over my laptop. She is a demanding dominant and I'm happy to serve her, to focus my energies around meeting her needs. I let the rest of the world slip away while she nurses from my breast. There is a sense of freedom in the experience, and I feel whole and complete in this energy exchange.

This feeling is not foreign to me. For the past six years, I've served her father as his submissive, lover, partner, and now the mother of his child. Ironically, my dedication to my child and my partner is what has made sitting down to write this essay the most challenging. My identity is complex—an interweaving of queer, masochist, rope slut, sex worker, control freak, loving partner, and mother. Within these carefully constructed labels, in order to find my true self, I must give in. I must allow myself to be taken over, not just to fall deep down the rabbit hole but to jump, to fly, to dive in with knowledge.

To be the truest form of myself, I leap into a world of submission.

I am a multifaceted woman with dominant and submissive tendencies, a wide range of desires for sensation play, and a need to play out different societal and animalistic roles in a safe environment with my partner. Sex is primal and has a magical, energetic rhythm to it—a pulse that you find in yourself or that passes between two or more persons. There are many ways to play with that pulse, that energy, both physically and psychologically. That pulse can be exchanged with great precision and control or it can knock you off your feet like a tidal wave.

> *Submission is instinctively serving my dominant, without effort, without being noticed or drawing attention.*

Submission caters to my Virgo love of control and precision. Submission fulfills me, in the eroticism of lists and charts, in the satisfaction of completing a task. Submission penetrates me deeply with the pleasure of rules to obey and jobs well done. Submission is falling into a Zen space of control: constructing my being as an instrument of use and pleasure, allowing energy to flow through me, reprogramming the fibers of my being to reflect the desires of my dominant. Submission is instinctively serving my dominant, without effort, without being noticed or drawing attention. It's all about the details and serving another, not indulging in one's own sexual impulses. It's a delicious mix of cerebral and visceral sexuality, of control and instinct, of pleasure and selflessness.

To submit to my dominant is to serve my dominant, to pleasure him, to obey protocol, and to serve as a useful tool in the completion of tasks. Submitting is making his life and household run more smoothly as well as providing entertainment and pleasure. When I submit to my dominant, I serve his erotic desires and fulfill mine; in practice, it might be as simple as walking behind my dominant and to his right side, fetching tea and preparing it the way he likes it, and never allowing his water glass to become less than half full at dinner. Or it could manifest as standing or kneeling rather than using a chair at dinner, a party, or on the subway. These small acts of submission enveloped in our day-to-day activities can fill my being with erotic energy and a sense of connectedness and commitment to each other.

In our D/s relationship, we have a contract and basic protocol rules. We have different levels of protocol: basic everyday protocol, high protocol, and, if need be, levels in between. One rule in our agreement states: "I will not use furniture, unless my dominant has given me permission or if abiding by this rule would inconvenience or make others around me uncomfortable." (I would not stand or kneel at a restaurant or cafe if I was there without my dominant or at a meeting where it would be inappropriate.) The rules in our contract help form the structure of our D/s relationship, and its creation is entirely unique to us. We understand that agreements can change based on the individuals' needs, which change over time, and we allow time on a regular basis to review our agreement to see what is working for each of us and what isn't. If something isn't working, we change it.

Sometimes, our D/s is incorporated into sex. I recall sitting at dinner at a four-star restaurant with my Sir. He ordered dessert for us, and as the waitress left the table he handed me a vibrator.

"Take this and get yourself off before our desert arrives, slut."

"Yes, Sir."

I took the vibrator underneath the white tablecloth, under my dress, and up my slit, until it rested next to my clit. The buzzing vibrator was barely audible over the espresso machine in the back. I worked my way up to climax and quietly asked, "Sir, may I come?"

"Yes, you may come."

"Thank you, Sir."

Other times, D/s manifests when my Sir enforces an order, like denying me orgasms. I remember one business trip where I would be in Detroit for a week, and my Dominant ordered me not to masturbate during the trip. I was so incredibly turned on by the fact that I wasn't allowed to touch myself that I nearly came simply by the denial of my masturbation privilege.

If my Dominant and I are engaging in sadomasochism,

I usually find myself in the role of a sensation-hungry lover or the submissive. If we are playing in an SM dynamic as lovers, I'm permitted to make eye contact. With each strike, we breathe together. It can be brutal and bloody, orgasmic and intimate all at the same time. If we're engaged in SM in a D/s protocol, I will not make eye contact and simply accept the energy of a whip or cane and allow it to flow through me without releasing moans of pleasure. I am only permitted to verbalize gratitude and respect, unless I am granted permission to come. In my role as a submissive, it's important for me to keep composure and always do my best to serve the needs of my Dominant, according to the terms of our D/s agreement, above my own impulses.

I was once performing in an on-camera scene with my Dominant and another woman. Her punishment for some indiscretion, which I now can't remember, was for her to watch as I took her caning for her. I knelt before my love, face forward, eyes focused ahead, arms behind my back, and took each strike with complete composure, only releasing breath and uttering a gracious "One. Thank you, Sir. Two. Thank you, Sir," until we reached 20 strikes. The girl stared at me crying and baffled by what she had just seen; she was puzzled to witness my intense composure to such a severe whipping and the deep level of submission I demonstrated.

In my relationship with my Dominant, he is my primary partner. But during the nearly six years of our relationship, I have petitioned for sexual and kinky relationships outside our own with agreed-upon partners. I once petitioned to be lent to a queer couple, a femme and a trans guy, for submissive service including domestic chores. The femme was the alpha Dominant in the relationship (both were dominant over me, but the femme Dominant was at the top of our hierarchy). After a decadent dinner in which I followed high-protocol standards (only speaking when spoken to, fetching jackets, pulling out chairs, opening the door) and serviced the couple sexually, I was ordered to the kitchen. A huge pile of dishes sat in the sink.

The two sat down at the kitchen table, postsex and orgasm, a bit disheveled, sipping on tea in their boxers, lingerie, and robes.

"Get to work, slut," Mistress ordered.

Naked and exhilarated in my submissive state, I got to work on the filthy dishes.

Mistress looked up drowsily from her tea and gifted me with her praise. "Such a good little submissive, slut. You are doing such a good job at those dishes. Jay, go get my whip."

Her partner returned with her whip and Mistress whipped my flesh, which was already marked from what had preceded in the bedroom that evening. As Mistress welted my skin with her whip, her fingers teasing my cunt every so often between strikes, and her partner sat at the kitchen table sipping his tea with a devilish grin, I felt absolute euphoric bliss in my service. It was one of those moments of clarity in which I feel that I am exactly where I am supposed to be, full of purpose and with

> **The grace and dignity with which a submissive accepts a punishment is just as important as the manner in which you conduct yourself in daily service.**

an internal stillness that exists only in absolute surrender.

Submission is a gift of full surrender to another person. It's the removal of ego and self-indulgence. When I engage in a heavy D/s scene, I picture myself as a hollow cane of bamboo: I allow energy to flow through me, keeping complete focus and attention to my surroundings on my Dominant, without drawing attention to myself. It requires being aware of the rhythm of life around me, life in my scene, and how I play into that rhythm, that cacophony of sound. For example, the sound of a key in the door cues me to remove my panties and kneel into slave position with arms folded behind my back. The sound of the shower's running water instinctively starts me calculating how long that sound will last before Sir exits the shower and I enter with a fresh folded towel. The sound of the whistling kettle activates my anticipation to prepare Sir's tea. The whistling kettle, the shower water, and the key in the door are just as kinky to my auditory senses as the sound of the flogger coming into impact with my grateful flesh, the whisk of a cane, the yelp of other submissives, and the cries of orgasmic pleasure that surround us in public dungeons. It is humbling to serve, to give in, without ego, mindful and focused.

But as submissives, we are human. We will make mistakes, and if we choose to disobey or act in a disrespectful manner, we will be punished. The grace and dignity with which a submissive accepts a punishment is just as important as the manner in which you conduct yourself in daily service. It may be even more important.

I remember one instance when I allowed my emotions

to get the better of me during a D/s scene with my Sir. Sir told me that because of a production schedule, he would have to work late on our anniversary, which was in a few weeks. This personal matter affected me as my Sir's lover, not as his submissive. I ran off from the scene in a huff and committed a cardinal sin in D/s: I took off my own collar. The collar is a symbol of dedication to our D/s relationship as well as a symbol of honor and respect reflecting my commitment to the BDSM community. In losing my composure and removing my collar, I was not only disrespecting my Sir but also acting as a disgrace to our community. Therefore my Sir decided that my punishment needed to be a public penance.

I treaded behind Sir in shame. I wished I could disappear and was thankful for the inviting darkness that the blindfold brought. I was led downstairs to a dungeon and placed on a suspended table; it was disorienting and difficult to balance on it without my sight. On all fours, presenting my ass, I awaited my punishment—rope biting around my chest, under my arms, pressed up against my rib cage, attempting to take over my breath and lead me into submission.

I felt floggers, paddles, hands, straps, belts, clamps, clothespins, and mouths. I gently cooed, "Thank you, Sir" and "Thank you, Ma'am." I heard later that a line had formed; everyone wanted their turn. I changed positions, presenting my chest, my pussy, rotating to give onlookers a better view. I stood in difficult stress positions, squatting, balancing—all blindfolded. My head was spinning, chasing after the texture of voices in the room. I heard people negotiating with Sir. As he handed me over to the next participant, one politely asked me, "Could I go harder?"

"If it pleases you, Sir."

Another said, "You seem like such a good girl. What could you possibly have done to deserve this punishment?"

"I'm not at liberty to say, Sir. I'm sorry, Sir."

I followed the words like light, like butterflies. I let the sensation wipe through me at the hands of seasoned leathermen and Dominants and newbies who were shy and nervous. You would have thought they were the ones under the whip.

I could feel a community around me—young and old, SMers, experimenters, and swingers. Each with a different stroke, a different touch. I was polite and grateful to them for taking part in my punishment.

Sir approached, whispering in my ear. "Just one more and I'll take you home."

"Thank you, Sir."

This swing was familiar. The cane struck my ass. I could feel the area of my flesh start to harden after repeated impact, and I could tell my skin had already started to bruise from hours of punishment. But I welcomed this touch. His touch.

"Count and show me you're sorry," he said.

"One. I'm sorry, Sir. Please, Sir, forgive me."

"Two. Sir, I'm so very sorry, Sir, I will be more mindful of my behavior, Sir."

"Three. Sir, I'm sorry, Sir. I will only show the greatest of respect to us and our protocol, Sir."

I felt tired and broken. Worn down but at the same time fulfilled. I felt an unselfish pleasure from a job well done.

"You did good tonight, Maddie. I'm very proud of you. You made a lot of people very happy."

"Thank you, Sir."

Sex-positive feminism embraces the entire range of human sexuality and is based on the idea that sexual freedom is an essential component of women's freedom. BDSM is based on power and sensation play with a strong emphasis on communication and consent. I validate my own desires through the act of submission while simultaneously taking control of and embracing my sexuality. I have had to fight for my sexuality and identity, and I educate others around me about it. My personal has always been political. The aggressiveness with which I embrace my queer identity has translated to aggressiveness in claiming my submission.

Why is it fascinating and stimulating to engage in power exchange? We are breaking the rules. As queers, feminists, kinky persons, and sexual outlaws, we have always broken the rules. We go outside designated sexual norms as we search for connection, community, and fulfillment in our sexual lives and identities. Our sexual selves were not handed to us—we had to create them. We disassemble traditional power structures put in place by social norms only to reassemble them to use as our own sex toys.

Submissives are often strong and powerful women and men who wish to set aside or give their power to another person. Submissives are willing to make themselves vulnerable and open to experiences. We serve and give something back to both our community and to the one(s) we serve. Our service and education can result in both personal growth and community development. We submit to better the lives of others and, in doing so, our submission enriches our own lives.

In a fantasy world, Sir and I would exist 24/7 in an erotically charged nonstop BDSM scene. But this is reality—and thank goodness it is! It would be boring and not nearly as special to me if submission were a constant. It is difficult to fully appreciate the calm without a healthy amount of chaos. Besides, Sir and I lead very hectic lives, and between work and our newborn baby girl, it's not possible for us to constantly maintain that dynamic of our relationship on a 24/7 basis. Instead we plan scenes or play dates. Or we find ways to work our D/s dynamic into our everyday lives. I welcome those moments like a breath of fresh air between diaper changes, breast-feedings, sexuality workshops, and business meetings. After six years together, my partner and I have found what works for us. And this is what works for us. We are able to be loving partners to each other, passionate lovers, cuddle buddies, and coparents to our daughter, all as we engage in a Dominant/submissive scene.

Sometimes it's just for a moment, something as simple as Sir pulling my hair and bringing me to my knees before he leans down, kisses me on the crown of my head, and whispers, "I love you, slut." Or me saying, "I love you, Sir" before we head out to work. Sometimes that is all the time we have. But it only takes a moment. It's a subtle shift of power, an opening of my being, slipping into that quiet stillness of perfection and tranquillity. It's a state of Zen submission.

The space I go to when I'm in a position of submission is

a meditative state. When painting or writing, I find myself going into a similar state. I have to step out of the way to give in to the creative energy. It's a state of pure connection, complete focus, and the clarity discovered in letting go. I find it by riding waves of energy that flow through me with each impact from a heavy flogger or sting of a singletail. I find it in the precision and mindfulness with which I complete a task for my Sir. To sink into subspace, I allow my day, my life, my identity outside that moment, outside that scene, to slip into the background, and I offer myself as a vessel for the energy exchange between me and my Dominant.

CHAPTER 15

ENHANCING MASOCHISM: HOW TO EXPAND LIMITS AND INCREASE DESIRE

PATRICK CALIFIA

It was the third SM play party I had ever attended. Since I was one of the organizers, it was up to me (and my cohost) to get things started, even though I was barely more experienced at group sex than most of the guests. That lovely lady (let's call her Fanny) was gracious enough to let me drag her into the center of the room and tie her up on all fours. She was a slender redhead with Celtic knots tattooed on her shoulders. The brightly entwined lines morphed into plants and fantastical animals as the design spilled onto her upper arms. She had long, very curly red hair, so she looked like a Raphaelesque angel you had divested of its robe and got ass-up and begging for cock. Like magic, as soon as we took off some of our clothes, everybody else formed couples and triads and got out their toys.

Fanny really, really, really wanted me to put my biggest strap-on in her ass. I did preliminary play with my fingers, an ass plug, and my second-biggest dildo. I massaged her, talked dirty to her, slipped lube into her butt, and played with her nipples. But her ass would only open so far. We had reached a plateau.

My pervy little angel was whispering something. Given the volume of the music and other players, the only thing I could hear was "Please, Sir." I leaned forward, but I couldn't get close enough to her head to decipher the whole message while I was manipulating a slender vibrator in her butt.

"Speak up!" I finally roared, letting a little of my frustration show in my voice.

"Get my belt!" she shouted, matching my volume. Apparently she was feeling a bit more frustrated than I was.

A passerby was kind enough to find her jeans and tug her simple leather belt out of the loops. I put down the vibes and plugs and dildos and picked up the supple length of that ordinary article of clothing. Suddenly it seemed vested with power and fear, an implement that might help us cross the line into a new realm of experience. I doubled it up and smacked her with it, drawing a broad red stripe across her pale, shapely ass, increasing the force until she was shuddering and dragging on the ropes. She had told me that she liked pain, but I didn't really get it until I saw her clawing at the leather tabletop, having what looked and sounded like an orgasm.

After that, we had no trouble getting my fat, 10-inch cock into her ass. She was as relaxed as could be. And if she did begin to tense up, all I had to do was trail the belt down her buttocks, pressing gently on her welts, to make her sigh and melt into me. It was a grand fuck, one of my first experiences with combining pain and pleasure, doing a scene that looked vanilla but most certainly was not.

Would this technique work with anybody? No. You have to start with at least some of the hardwiring for masochism. If you do have that hardwiring, should you be expected to stand up and get bull-whipped for an hour, with no warm-up, to entertain a crowd at a leather community fund-raiser for breast cancer? Only if you are an exceptionally heavy player and such an exhibitionist that nothing matters but the spectators. But can you perhaps learn to take a bit more, and then a bit more, to please a lover and yourself? Yes.

SOME DEFINITIONS

In this article I use the term *masochism* to refer to the desire and the ability to become aroused and perhaps even climax while experiencing sensations that other people avoid. Although I talk about pain and discomfort, it should be understood that once a masochist is aroused and in a state of surrender to these intense sensations, they are not experiencing the kind of pain that someone who is ill or traumatized feels when they are shocked by how torturous it can be to have a body. I also want to note that there are masochists who seek out pain even if it does not arouse them; willingly tolerating hurt can have a number of positive results, which will be clear a little further on.

Unfortunately, the stigma of the label *masochism* has been perpetuated by sex-negative doctors, psychologists, and other mental health "professionals" whose vocabularies lack precision. So-called experts get away with claiming that masochism is unhealthy because they use the term loosely to describe other types of human behavior as well. Patients who stay in violent relationships, allow themselves to be exploited by employers or family members, can't take control over their own lives, or harm themselves physically and emotionally are referred to as exhibiting masochism. Most of these people haven't got a kinky bone in their bodies. Yet people who enjoy being spanked, whipped, pinched, bitten, etc. because it gives them an erotic rush and makes them feel closer to their partners are also called masochists.

This flawed logic has resulted in the diagnosis "sexual masochism" appearing in the *Diagnostic and Statistical Manual-IV TR (DSM-IV-TR),* the industry standard for mental-health bureaucracy. "Sexual sadism" is in there, too. You can't write a case report, create a treatment plan, or (most importantly) bill an insurance company without using the *DSM*'s nomenclature of supposed dysfunction.

Is there any objective proof that people who get wet during a spanking are also getting ripped off financially, intimidated by bullies, anorexic, being battered, or likely to engage in self-mutilation? No. And there never will be, because we are conflating two separate categories of human experience. One is a sexual identity or experience; the other is a state of disenfranchisement, oppression, traumatization, or self-hatred. People consent to the former; they wish they could escape the latter. The earliest attempts to educate mental-health professionals about BDSM focused on the fact that this was a sexual style based on consent and negotiation. These were pleasurable acts committed by adults who chose to enjoy kinky sex. This message reached a certain number of people. But it is very difficult to overturn generations of fear and disgust. For many "experts" whose credentials allowed them to pronounce on our mental health (or sickness), the fact that people would consent to do these things became proof that BDSM players had to be mentally ill. If you weren't crazy, this reasoning goes, you wouldn't want to do these things or agree to have them done to you. For therapists who are judgmental about sexual variation, the fact that someone would consent to wearing a pair of nipple clamps or having their face slapped just proves that they are indeed sick and unable to distinguish between healthy and unhealthy experiences. And the person who does such awful things to them is a monster.

For alleged social scientists to judge human sexuality this way is embarrassing. The assumption that variant sexualities are mental illnesses has more to do with conservative religious values than it does with objective observation. If a mental state or human behavior is unhealthy, we ought to be able to demonstrate that it makes that person unhappy, interferes with their ability to give and receive love, prevents them from setting goals that give them a sense of fulfillment, and injures their health. It's not enough to say BDSM is sick or crazy because most people don't do it. Most people don't become concert pianists or Olympic athletes, either. These are individual dreams of excellence that cause people to devote a great deal of time and effort to perfecting their abilities. If you took away the opportunity to compete in their chosen field, these "minority members" would be devastated. Does that prove they are addicted or coerced into loving classical music or diving from high places? You can see how this line of thinking breaks down if we ask some reasonable questions.

This is not to say that BDSMers (or our relationships) are always happy and strong. Our community has its share of people who are mean-spirited or manipulative or crackers. Some of us find romantic love and lots of sex with ease; others experience higher levels of loneliness and unsatisfied desire. But this is simply the human condition. It's okay for us to be imperfect. We struggle, like anyone else, to figure out what sort of relationships are ethical or will meet our needs, how to communicate unwelcome information to a partner, whether to let a conflict result in separation or rededication to the relationship. That doesn't prove that we are sick or crazy. As long as we are conscious of our own and others' well-being, and striving to contribute to that, we are on a good path and we don't need to engage in harmful self-criticism.

AN ALTERNATIVE VIEW OF MASOCHISM

How many times have you heard someone say, "Pain is a warning that our bodies are in danger"? It sounds like a truism. But, like most assumptions, it deserves a closer look. While pain can be a symptom of disease or injury, human beings have always sought to control their reaction to pain. If we couldn't tolerate at least some discomfort, sadness, anxiety, or less-than-wonderful physical states, how would any of us get through an ordinary day—much less deal with hard work or a chronic illness?

For millions of years, people have deliberately constructed painful situations and faced them to obtain a number of different benefits. In some societies, painful ordeals or body modification mark an individual's transition from childhood to adulthood. Obtaining spiritual guidance has often required a sacrifice, to prove the seriousness of one's intent and create an altered state that allows communication between this world and other realms. Consciously choosing to suffer discomfort has resulted in the acquisition of wisdom, experiencing divine rapture, obtaining healing, and locating and killing meat for the cooking pot. Whether the goal is mundane or transcendental, the ability to use our hearts and minds to convince our bodies to continue to function while we are aching (or worse) is the hallmark of courage, loyalty, and strength.

One of the most painful physical events a human being can endure is the birth of a child. Are women "masochistic" because they endure pregnancy and birth?

The rituals and other trials I described above are not examples of sexual masochism. But they highlight the physiological reasons why it's possible for us to get aroused by pain. When our bodies feel stress, they autonomously produce chemicals that help us cope. We may pant, bringing extra oxygen into our bodies. Adrenaline, endorphins, and natural narcotics flood our nervous system. Euphoria and agony are next-door neighbors—you can't break that paradoxical connection. And if you are not willing to tolerate contradictions and paradoxes, human behavior will never make much sense to you.

Postindustrial Western societies romanticize sex. To some extent, this is good. I wouldn't want to go back to a time when premarital sex hardly existed, women had no sexual autonomy, and marriages were arranged by the couple's families. Falling in love is a good reason to be together, even if its initial intensity can rarely be sustained forever.

We've come to expect a level of intimacy and understanding or rapport, especially in the first stages of sexual experience, that very few lovers can sustain. Some women's first experience of intercourse is easy; others feel varying degrees of twinginess or even a stab of pain when the hymen is broken. But even after that inconvenience is eliminated, it takes some practice for two bodies (especially two bodies of dissimilar gender) to create a mutual rhythm of lovemaking. Being able to tolerate discomfort or even get turned on by it may be one of the things that helps us put up with each other long enough to get better at providing pleasure.

> *Euphoria and agony are next-door neighbors— you can't break that paradoxical connection.*

On an online message board for kinky women, a conversation took place about why experiencing pain makes some women get wet. In less civilized times, getting hurt might be a signal that sexual assault was going to occur. One or two of them speculated that this reflex might have helped their gender survive rape.

I have no idea whether most women or only a handful get physically excited by roughness or pain. Even if this reaction occurs, it does *not* justify violence against women. Rape is evil because it involves using another's body as if they were an object, ignoring the person inside and their response to it. Most of the time, rape is an unpleasant and squalid experience that has no pleasurable content. But even if rape results in an orgasm for the victim, I assert that it is as evil to give someone an orgasm against their will as it is to fuck them while preventing them from coming.

We like to think of pleasure as good and pain as bad, but the Shadow side of us sees through that simplistic thinking. I have seen more hatred expressed in an act of vanilla sex than I could believe, and I have seen inexpressible tenderness while one partner bled and the other inhaled their pain like the bouquet of a rare wine.

WHO'S THERE?

This "big picture" stuff is fun to think about, discuss, and research. But it's a little too abstract to help two people who want to branch out in the bedroom and get into some daunting activities. How can you make your socially unacceptable, thigh-squeezing, nubby-nippled, ball-tightening dreams come true?

It helps to give some preliminary thought to the psychology of both top and bottom. When I do workshops on BDSM role playing, I like to give participants four different scales that they can use to rate themselves, for masochism, sadism, submission, and dominance. Each of these qualities is independent of the others. I've met dominant masochists and submissive sadists, for example.

Why someone is going to inflict or accept a sensation is as important as who will be playing each part. A masochist may be willing to pretend they are submissive just so they can get whipped till they cry. Without the catharsis of a good workout on a regular basis, the masochist gets cranky and sluggish and depressed. As long as they are black-and-blue, they are perky and industrious. You may get more out of a masochist if you dispense with courtesies such as waiting at the table or picking up heavy things and letting them tell you which implements they adore, which ones they laugh at, and which ones strike terror into their hearts. I've seen joyous and amazing pain play that had not a shred of role playing in it. (This does not mean, by the way, that a masochist cannot be quite loyal and helpful to you, if only because you see and value a side of them that the world despises.)

A submissive may not like pain at all unless it is presented as a service that they are required to perform for the master or mistress. It is the submissive's obligation to provide service and give pleasure—to yield and submit to a higher will. Pain can be administered as a symbol of ownership. "I can do this to you because you belong to me, and you will take it because it excites and relaxes me."

If you don't know where you fit in this complex picture, don't worry about it too much. It can take a lot of experience to figure out your own psychic twists and turns. Very few of us are exclusively top or bottom. If there wasn't at least a crumb of masochism in the sadist, how could he or she understand what they are asking the bottom to do? Not to mention the fact that people's needs often change as life changes them.

Even if you know your pain tolerance can be rated on the heavy end of the scale, be prepared for its fickleness. There will be nights when the paddle that you worshipped last time is just too evil to be borne. Remember that the point of doing a scene is how it makes you feel, not the techniques or toys being used. A good top understands this, and won't throw a hissy if you need to be beaten with a terry-cloth bathrobe tie.

I hope it won't completely confuse the issue to say that not all pain trips require a top and a bottom. Some people who create ordeals view themselves as spiritual guides or assistants; they don't want a romantic relationship. I've heard hot stories of two competitive bottoms who got together to see who would use their safeword first. And, during those periods of drought when the bars and parties and clubs seem populated by toads and trolls, the self-infliction of sexy pain is a very nice adjunct to masturbation. Who could you trust more than yourself?

SET AND SETTING

The terms *set* and *setting* were coined by Timothy Leary to describe factors that determine the experience of ingesting psychedelic drugs. It is useful to consider these factors because they influence the emotional content of an event, whether it is theater, long-distance running, or therapy. *Set* has to do with the participants' mind-set, the internal processes that can either enhance or destroy pleasure. *Setting* refers to the location where the event takes place—what you see, smell, touch, hear, and feel around you.

These factors are highly individual. If the steps I suggest don't sound effective for you, you are the best judge of that. But at least I can give you some specific ideas that have proven their worth for me and other players. This can help you pin down your own experimental parameters. And after every session, it's a good idea to discuss what did and didn't work, with an eye to brainstorming new possibilities for erotic play. If you must give your partner negative feedback, express it with tenderness, and surround your misgivings with praise for what did work. Both top and bottom make themselves equally vulnerable in a session. If the only thing you can come up with is a barrage of criticism or inflated demands, the two of you are probably incompatible.

Take a look at the space where the scene is going to happen. Do enough preparation so that the two of you can be spontaneous. Everything you are going to need should be in the room. Leave the room if you must, but be aware you are opening the oven and letting some of the heat out. When you return, you'll need to back up a little and build up to the point you reached when the two of you broke connection.

The room needs to be clean—well, for most fetishes. Toys ought to be organized, in good repair, and accessible. Lube and safe-sex barriers should be in clear view. Rope ought to be untangled, clean, inspected for weaknesses, and laid out so it won't turn into a snarl the minute the top touches it. If you are going to play with locking devices, make sure there are extra keys, and that both of you know where they are.

Think of this as foreplay. You can start getting excited by your own sexiness, and by anticipating your partner's presence. Touching your toys and disinfecting a play surface is like caressing your own body. Your energy, sense of purpose, or consciousness starts gathering into a focus on Eros.

Before you play, ask yourself what makes you feel alluring and powerful. (I am including bottoms here because you need your own strength. The session comes from you as much as, if not more than, from the top.) Take the time and trouble to dress up, even if you are only wearing a beautiful collar or a badass pair of boots. Get enough rest and eat a healthy meal a couple of hours before you play.

I'm going to assume that you've already been educated about how to negotiate a scene, get any needed consent, choose a safeword, etc. I'm also going to assume that you know your way around the toys or equipment you will use. This is an article about pain play in general; describing every single technique is beyond my scope. *Never* pretend to have experience that you lack. There is honor only in being honest about this and making sure you get trained to an expert level.

Unless you are the Ice Queen escorting your latest paramour to your frigid palace, I recommend taking the bottom into a warm room. Loose, relaxed muscles are going to accept building sensations more easily. I also suggest taking away one of your bottom's senses, if only for a little while. Using a blindfold or gag is your first demand for control over their body. Can they let go and graciously accede to allowing you to orchestrate their experience?

Take the time to verbally or visually remind the two of you (or your birthday party guests) who it is you are manifesting in this fantasy. In what time or place are you encountering each other? You can do a simple breathing exercise to get grounded in the present. Or perhaps you've constructed an elaborate story with chapters and verses. This provides a meaningful context for pain.

During some sessions, the reason for the infliction of pain is elicited from the bottom while they are under duress ("You're hurting me because I'm a dirty pig!" or "You are giving me pain to push me out of my body, so I can fly free.") In the past, I have said that it is the top's responsibility to determine what each action means and share that significance with the bottom. But I have come to see that finding this underlying meaning is really a joint project. It may be a conspiracy that can be verified by silently meeting each other's eyes, or it may be a sudden revelation that has to be shouted or whispered aloud. You may find the answer in your own heart or see it emerging in the shape of your partner's face. It can be an old friend, an enemy, or a complete surprise.

Arousing the bottom is an important first step, unless you are playing with a rare and wonderful creature who needs pain to get aroused. Give your partner a brief massage. Highlight the genitals but don't give them too much attention. You want to create anticipation by teasing. If the bottom has a favorite toy that already gets them going, why not begin with that. Proceed from the familiar to the unfamiliar. Bondage can be very helpful. It allows the bottom to feel contained and secure, and gives them something to pull on when things get exciting.

I dearly love to mix sexual stimulation with gradually increasing levels of pain. I also want to keep the bottom awake and responsive, so I won't use the same implement for too long. If I am whipping someone, I switch between implements that go "thud" and skinny, flexible tools that sting. As blood rises to the surface of the skin, it becomes more sensitive; sometimes running your fingertips or a piece of fur over the skin is exquisite, almost too much so. I also like to vary dry skin versus wet during a whipping or spanking. Generally, wet skin is more sensitive.

Alternating with the bad behavior, I am kissing the bottom, stroking their body, locating various erogenous zones, and titillating them. I want them to need my touch. Winning pleasure is a reward for enduring or enjoying a low level of pain. Be patient with this type of training. It can take several sessions before you begin to see the bottom opening up and allowing you to do more and more. Trust can't always be built in one session.

A bottom who needs safety before they can take down their walls will appreciate being asked how they are doing and reminded that this is all within their control. (It is a common joke among tops who enjoy electrical play that if you give the bottom a control box, they will smartly turn up the dial to levels that were not allowed when the control rested in the top's hand.) You might think that safety is a universal requirement for all masochists, but I have found instead that a certain amount of realism may be necessary to unlock an erotic response to higher levels of pain. If you really are a captive, you know you will have to take more than the person who is playing at being a captive.

Fear is the most powerful obstacle to building up a tolerance for and erotic response to pain. It may sound corny, but I love to recite the Bene Gesserit rite about pain from the *Dune* novels. Get the bottom to pay attention to what is really going on, right now, rather than their exaggerated and panicky image of what might happen to them. I find that if I can get a bottom to stick with me for the first 20 minutes or so, a whip or a fistful of clothespins suddenly gets a whole lot easier to take. That's because naturally occurring chemicals are beginning to hit the bloodstream, turning "pain" into "wheeee"!

If you are able to feel energy around yourself and your partner, remind them that you want to link the two of you together. I have found that it often works to create a vocal circuit between me and my partner. When I hurt them, they can open their mouth and by panting or making a noise pass the pain on to me. I take the pain, turn it into pleasure, and push it back into them. (I may be pushing other things into them as well, dirty lowlife that I am.) It's amazing how often people will experience exactly what you tell them to feel. If you have a certain destination in mind, take the bottom there, one blow or pinch or slap at a time.

If you are playing with a submissive rather than a pure masochist, you can use service-oriented psychology to build tolerance for pain. As I said earlier, the submissive wants to be possessed and yield to another person; they want to be of service. They will take pain if you make it their job to take it. The pain becomes one item on a menu of conduct or sacrifices that you, the master or mistress, demand because it pleases you. Pain becomes a way to demonstrate your control over him or her. But this may not occur to your submissive unless you spell it out. People tend to get confused during play—they are in an altered state. So speak slowly and use simple words if you feel you are not getting through.

CONSENSUAL NONCONSENT

For some bottoms, the object of painful techniques is to be out of control. They do not want a cooperative, mutually negotiated scenario, but rather a nonconsensual fantasy and a fair amount of force. Restraints will have to be strong and escape-proof. They need to struggle and suffer until they reach a phase of liberation or release. They may want to be "broken." I urge newer players especially to proceed carefully. The emotional consequences of a session can last long after the toys have been put away. So be cautious of a scene this heavy—do you want to take care of a bottom who has lost their will to you? And if you are a bottom seeking a scene of this nature, please take responsibility for your own feelings and needs. It is unethical to expect a top to take on a larger role in your life than they wish to take. Do not engage in harassment or stalking! If you know you will be vulnerable after a heavy scene, arrange care for yourself before you play, so you don't crash when you are all alone and have no resources to keep you connected to the human race. As sweet as those endorphins are, losing them is a wicked crash.

Many of us associate pain with punishment, and fantasy punishment scenarios abound in BDSM play. There are lots of teachers who paddle unruly students, daddies who have to put little girls (age 32) in the corner, guards who flog convicts who tried to escape, etc. Punishment can put the top and bottom in an adversarial dynamic. If this disturbs you, you may want to require the bottom to admit that they deserve the punishment, and aim the scene toward getting them to feel more attached to you. By beating them, you are driving them toward the safe cage of your possessiveness. Or you may find, as a top, that when you are in a certain wicked mood, you don't want to make nice, you just want to kick the shit out of somebody who knows they belong on the floor.

In most scenes that include significant levels of discomfort, the bottom will reach a plateau. There are a number of ways to deal with a bottom who says they can't take any more. One possibility is to take them at their word and end the scene, praising them for what they were able to do. If you feel that they are capable of more and may be disappointed later if they give up, you may want to simply take a break and see if some comfort and protein can screw up their courage once more. If the bottom told you there were certain things they wanted to experience, and the two of you haven't made that happen yet, they may be motivated to dig a little deeper if you remind them of what their masochistic ambitions were prior to play.

> *Sometimes people cannot willingly go where they need to go—they have to be taken there. This is a controversial observation, and most people will want to steer clear of it.*

Sometimes people cannot willingly go where they need to go—they have to be taken there. This is a controversial observation, and most people will want to steer clear of it. For most of us, it is safest to stick with the zone of play where we have clear, uncomplicated consent. It's a dicey proposition for a top to ignore a bottom's pleas and continue to hurt them until they yield. You wind up manifesting a great deal of the Shadow, and you'll feel quite a backlash from that.

Once upon a time, play without limits or safewords was very common in the gay men's leather community. A bottom was expected to do some research on a master before approaching him. Did you really want it, or not? If you made a bid for his attention and he took you home, you were supposed to make yourself available for whatever he liked to do. He was God, and you were dirt. Whining later was seen as sissy bullshit. If you whined, no top would touch you—you were an unreliable coward who might make secret and sacred things public to the authorities.

I appreciate the modern, pansexual kinky community's desire to keep BDSM safe, sane, and consensual (as the old slogan goes). But I sometimes think we have allowed the pendulum to swing too far in the direction of predictable scenes in which the top functions as an extra pair of hands for the bottom. While it can be a great deal of fun to help your bottom masturbate to their favorite things, is there not some way to make equal space for what the top wants? It is a double bind, being expected to exercise a dark and wonderful power while obsessing with the intricacies of the bottom's sensitivities, perpetually second-guessing them. A lot of the bottoms I meet nowadays seem terribly spoiled to me, and very unhappy, because they don't really want to be running things. More than a few good bottoms in our little world seem lost under the current mores. They long for the thrill of encountering the harsh will of an Other who is severe and powerful. Here's a story about this impasse.

I once participated in a whipping booth at a fund-raiser for the Operation Spanner defendants. (We were raising money for a small, private club of British leathermen who had been arrested and charged with assault for doing consensual SM with each other.) Prospective bottoms were allowed to pick any of several implements and specify the number of strokes and the level of intensity they desired. I was surprised how many eager novices lined up to see what it was all about. This seemed to be a safe way to try new toys and be just a bit of a masochist.

Toward the end of the event, after almost everyone had left, I was ready to pack it in. But one woman was very persistent. When I told her she would not be able to use the tickets she had purchased and offered her a refund, she was quite upset. She told me she had never been caned, she was terrified of it, but she felt so compelled to be caned that she was going out of her mind. She literally begged me to show her what it would be like to be out of control from pain.

So I bent her over the leather whipping bench, held her down with one hand on her lower back, and caned the bejesus out of her. She had asked for a dozen strokes and began to protest when we reached eight. "I have to insist on giving you what you asked for when you first talked to me," I told her, "because I think that is what you really want and need." So I hit her quite hard for the last four strokes, then added an additional one—"So you know that everything is not up to you. Sometimes the top will decide what you get."

She was dizzy when she straightened up, and beaming. So

proud of herself and grateful. She fell on my neck and hugged and kissed me. I even got a thank-you card from her years later. Sadly, in all that time, she had encountered no one who would help her over the hump by ignoring her pleas for mercy. What a waste of talent and thrills! Now, there was a potential masochist worth their salt.

But you can see how easily this scenario could have gone all pear-shaped, as our British colleagues would say. If I had been wrong in my assessment of her, she could very easily have come up from the table fighting mad, and justifiably so. She could have accused me of assaulting her. It certainly would have harmed my reputation (such as it is, poor sooty thing) and upset everyone who heard about it. We talk very little, regrettably, about how much the top needs to be able to trust the bottom. Buyer's remorse can ruin another player's life.

If it makes your crotch tingle to squeeze someone's balls until he protests, or take a sharp little blade to her inner thigh, or if you can't wait to get a blow job after you see the first bruises appear on a healthy pair of buns—well, you are by definition a sadist. The psychiatric experts pity masochists as self-harming fools. But they think sadists are dangerous. The *DSM-IV-TR* has some very silly things to say about sadists becoming rapists and killers.

The vulnerability of the masochist is plain. There they are, perhaps bound, heart pounding, dreading what is going to happen next, promising themselves that if they can just get through this one session they will never ask to be whipped/branded/clipped/pierced/squeezed/frozen/tattooed again. But what about the leather-clad bastard who is going to put this poor, naked person through hell? Never mind that the masochist begged and pleaded for it yesterday. The expense of the equipment, the time it took to locate a soundproof space and good bondage equipment, all this effort is seen as self-serving rather than an honest attempt to make the bottom's dreams come true.

NO-FAULT PLAY

It's so easy to make a mistake once play begins. People shut down and quit communicating. In semidarkness, a whip may land where it shouldn't. A game that was great fun two weeks ago is causing flashbacks tonight. The suspension equipment breaks, resulting in a painful fall, or a cane cracks in half and cuts someone. And yet everyone involved in these scenes had the best of intentions, and did everything within reason to be a good play partner.

This is why I recommend a no-fault attitude for BDSM players. As long as both partners respect each other, make a good-faith effort to abide by each other's limits, and are open to feedback, I think that missteps ought to be understood as part of the price you pay for being on the edge. Indifferent or bad experiences are there to teach us how to avoid them. A couple or group who have an accident ought to give and receive comfort, make up, and keep learning. It takes a lot of experience, and a certain amount of innate talent, to correctly assess and challenge the central nervous system. Luck is a factor as well!

If you take any of the above paragraphs as an excuse for

being lazy, negligent, or callous, well, you just ought to go to hell, that's all I have to say. And I'll probably be there to shovel some coal on the blaze.

ENOUGH, ALREADY!

In closing, let me bring up one more controversial fact. The heavier the scene, the more both partners experience weariness, anxiety, and aches and pains. It takes a lot of strength, grace, and stamina to work on someone's body for a prolonged period of time. If you are a switch or a top, what is your attitude toward your own pain tolerance? Do you disapprove of it or ignore it? Do you pretend it doesn't exist? Or do you work with it to build your own excitement? More than one dominatrix is wearing a pair of nipple clamps under her bustier to keep herself focused on her sniveling client. A famous domme author once referred to her extra-high heels as giving her a useful reservoir of irritability. I find it fascinating that in consensual BDSM, tops and bottoms and switches can all have a relationship with pain as a beloved friend and reward.

Some of my favorite play partners are tops who need a break. I am more than happy to anonymously provide a vacation for them at the other end of the whip. Every partner of mine is entitled to confidentiality. But because our community can be so stupid and judgmental about tops who get tired of always being the one to bark out the orders, I never even note the identities of these people in my journal. (As if anybody could ever read my handwriting.)

When a bottom whimpers and tells me they can't take any

more, I have been known to whip out a pair of needles and pierce my own nipples. While they watch. If I can take it, I ask, why can't they?

And that's the perfect place to stop. Because there's only so much you can learn from reading a book. Go outside and play.

CHAPTER 16

INSIDE THE MIND OF A SADIST

FIFTHANGEL

In the dungeon, we entered what Katie and I call "Thunderdome." Thunderdome is one of those large jungle gym–type things with hundreds of bars linked together to form a half dome. This particular one is rather immense and stands some 12 feet high—tall enough for suspension work. Katie very much enjoys being suspended upside down, so that was the plan for our night, though she had no idea what else I was going to do in this scene. Katie and I have been married for a few years now, and we do not use a safeword that enables her to stop a scene. Of course, if something is terribly wrong or very unsafe, she will bring it to my attention.

I started off by restraining her feet to a metal spreader bar that I had made. After her feet were clamped to the bar, I suspended her upside down from the top of the dome. I lashed her hands together behind her back with deep-red-colored hemp rope that she made for me. The rope is well used and scarred with bloodstains from prior scenes.

As with most times when I have sex with my wife, I did not have an organized plan. What happens is really a matter of what enters my head at the time, so my thoughts and actions are always subject to what she may say or do. For some reason, while I was binding her up, she moved in a direction I did not want. I said something to the effect of "Stop fucking moving." She instantly began to cry for fear that something unpleasant was going to follow. She would only have this type of reaction during a scene because, in the past, I have punished the part of the body that made the mistake. It keeps her thinking about what not to do. While she cried, I continued my bondage work.

Underneath her were chux pads (medical drop cloths the size of a medium bath towel) to keep the floor clean and collect anything that might come out of her. The vast dungeon was dimly lit in this area, which made clear vision a challenge. Nonetheless, I was able to see the shadows cast by her external jugular veins. Because she was dangling from her feet, the veins in her neck had become engorged with blood.

I felt her neck veins with the pad of my finger, which let her know I was going to draw blood. Because her adrenaline was elevated from the excitement of the scene and she was suspended upside down, I knew I had limited time to work before she might pass out. I placed two holes in one of her jugular veins with an 18-gauge needle. Blood began to squirt from her neck and onto the white chux, and slowly dripped down her face, pooling below her. My cock was very hard at this point and I wanted it inside her. Unfortunately, I hadn't thought that part all the way through beforehand—it was impossible with her upside down.

My next-best solution was to bring her to orgasm by licking and tasting her pussy. Her legs were spread apart and her waist was at the height of my face, so this worked out well. It did not take long for her to have an orgasm. Her body shuddered and withered against the restraints and even more blood oozed from her neck due to the increased pressure in her body from the orgasm. Okay, I thought, she had her fun. Now it's my turn.

DOMINANT, TOP, OR SADIST?

Later that evening and the next day, many people spoke to us about the scene and how hot it was. But what did they see? Was I being a Dominant? Many would agree that I was topping. Were there any elements of sadism? Viewing a scene from the outside, it can be difficult to see what the dynamics really are.

> *A Dominant, a Sadist, or a Top can wield a flogger, and by outward appearances they may appear the same; the difference is in the intent of the flogging, the receiver's perception, and what you can't see.*

I have fulfilled the roles of Dominant, Top, and Sadist at various times in my tenure in the world of BDSM. The names of these roles vary to suit the user; the language can be imprecise. Although you can assume multiple roles simultaneously,

I believe there are significant differences worth exploring. The emphasis of this piece will be sadism, since I feel it is the most complex, the least understood, and there are fewer examples of it in the kink community.

A Dominant, a Sadist, or a Top can wield a flogger, and by outward appearances they may appear the same; the difference is in the *intent* of the flogging, the receiver's perception, and what you can't see.

Top is an all-encompassing role; topping describes the *actions* performed by one person (the Top) on another (the bottom), like wielding the flogger. But topping does not describe *behavior*. Behavior is how a person conducts himself or interacts with the environment around him. In the case of flogging, a Top's intent is to flog the bottom, to create various sensations on the bottom's body. The flogging may be pleasurable for the bottom, even playful and fun. The Top may gain pleasure from the flogging, but not necessarily sexual pleasure. The key element is that these actions do not have to lead to sexual arousal or gratification for the Top or the bottom.

Dominance reflects a set of *behaviors* or a type of relationship. It is a dynamic where a power exchange takes place; the Dominant accepts control over another person (often, but not always, the submissive), and the submissive gives up control or power to the Dominant. Do not confuse giving up control with giving consent—everything we do is consensual. Dominance can be, but does not have to be, about sexual encounters or sexual gratification. Using flogging as an example again, a Dominant may employ flogging to communicate his control over the submissive's body, making the submissive bend to his will, achieving the same result as a Top. The Dominant gains personal satisfaction in accepting and exercising this control.

Sadism is a set of *behaviors* (or fantasies) involving the emotional or physical suffering of another that is sexually exciting to the Sadist. This is all about sexual gratification, nothing else. When a Sadist flogs someone, she wants them to suffer and be in pain at some point. Note that the pain and suffering are not sexually exciting to the bottom.

A Dominant becomes a Top or Sadist within a scene. A Dominant can be sadistic in a scene while he or she is topping. A Sadist does not have to be a Dominant in a scene, and vice versa. I would like to emphasize that dominance is a set of behaviors, not *physical actions*. As a supervisor in my career field, I have taken numerous behavioral tests, and in every case I was classified as "dominant"—an assessment that has nothing to do with my physical actions. Now, as a test subject for sadism, observe how hard my cock gets when my wife is in extreme pain and suffering.

A BRIEF HISTORY OF SADISM

I am most noted for my consensual sadistic behavior, and I have performed a great deal of research on the subject of sadism—not to understand my own behavior, but to understand its origins, its history, and the language involved, kind of like some sick behavioral family tree, I guess. So let's talk about sadism for a bit.

> The ravished girls were led away to marriage; their very shame made them more beautiful. And when one struggled hard against her captor, He carried her away in eager arms, And said: "Why spoil your pretty eyes by weeping? Your father took your mother, I take you!"
>
> —OVID[1]

In the eyes of the poet, the psychological shame of the girls made them more attractive and maybe even sexually aroused the onlookers. Unmistakably, when the girl struggled knowing she was going to have sex, possibly forcible sex, her captor was still happy. It is safe to say sex has been around a long time. Is it inconceivable that sexual gratification from the suffering of others has been around just as long?

The behavior that we know today as sadism has been around for thousands of years, but there wasn't a name for it until recently. Could it be that this was just normal, accepted behavior for the times? And how did this behavior, along with all the evil circumstance that ill-informed people associate with it, come to be known as sadism?

The vast majority of people in the BDSM community probably disagree with the definition of sadism as put forth in the medical literature. I will attempt to shed a favorable light on this subject by explaining the changes associated with the medical definition of sadism. It is my hope that you will agree, as evidenced by these changes, that it is no longer an evil sexual practice but can be an accepted sexual behavior.

Richard Freiherr von Krafft-Ebing (1840–1902), a German-

Austrian psychiatrist, adopted the term *sadism* for professional use in 1898; however, he first discussed the sexual nature of sadistic experiences in 1886, in *Psychopathia Sexualis*:

> The experience of sexual, pleasurable sensations (including orgasm) produced by acts of cruelty, bodily punishment afflicted on one's person or when witnessed in others, be they animals or human beings. It may also consist of an innate desire to humiliate, hurt, wound or even destroy others in order, thereby, to create sexual pleasure in ones self.[2]

By using the adjective *innate*, Krafft-Ebing shows he firmly believes one can be born a Sadist. I completely agree with this possibility; I often say I am just wired this way. Later definitions of sadistic behaviors put forth by the psychology community did not include Krafft-Ebing's original assertion that Sadists could derive sexual pleasure from watching others receiving acts of cruelty or bodily punishment.[3] This is especially important to me because I do become sexually aroused when watching a *scene* in which the bottom is suffering. Yet, I do not derive sexual pleasure while watching a fistfight or poking my patients with needles for blood draws.

Krafft-Ebing used the term *sadism* to describe a set of sexual behaviors, specifically the behaviors practiced and written about by the Marquis de Sade, a renowned French author who lived from 1740 to 1814. It is obvious the word *sadism* is derived from the name of de Sade himself as well as the French word *sadisme*. *Sadisme* appeared in an 1834 French dictionary written by lexicographer Pierre-Claude-Victor Boiste. Krafft-Ebing's original definition did not differentiate between consensual or nonconsensual acts. One can argue that his definition addresses nonconsensual behavior, as this is what the Marquis de Sade wrote about. The marquis's works included graphic descriptions of acts in which the "victim" (I put this in quotes because today we call them bottoms) was made to suffer, feel pain, and be humiliated, which resulted in the sexual gratification of the aggressor. For example:

> He bleeds both of her arms and would have her remain standing while her blood flows; now and again he stops the bleeding and flogs her, then he opens the wounds again, and this continues until she collapses. He only discharges when she faints.[4]

She raises a storm, criticizing their behavior toward her and describing it as unjust. *"'Were it just,' says the Duc, wiping his razor, 'it would surely fail to give us an erection.'"*[5]

> But the darling girl's pleas were worse than futile, for Dubourg, far from being disgusted by the spectacle of her suffering, actually savored it, delighted in it, thrived on it! Striking her once, twice, a third time, he fell madly on top of her and began nuzzling her bloody mouth.[6]

You may have heard the term *sexual sadism*. Given the fact that *sadism* was coined to explain a form of sexual gratification, many authorities believe it is redundant to say "sexual sadism," preferring simply "sadism."

Not only did the Marquis de Sade write about acts of sexual perversion, he apparently indulged in them. His most famous "victim" was Rose Keller. According to the court in which he was tried for his acts, de Sade picked up Rose Keller and took her to a home in Arcueil where he reportedly bound and flogged her. Due to the lack of physical evidence, it is not known whether de Sade raped her.

Among the numerous reports of his participation in orgies, one well-known account states that he hired four prostitutes to take part in an orgy that included a round of flogging during which everyone was flogged, including de Sade himself and his servant. It was this encounter for which the marquis was arrested for poisoning and sodomy. De Sade was accused of slipping something equivalent to Spanish fly into some aniseed sweets. (Rather than sexually arousing the prostitutes, it made them very sick.)

In 1898, Krafft-Ebing described sadistic behavior in sexual terms:

> The quality of sadistic acts is defined by the relative potency of the tainted individual. If potent, the impulse of the sadist is directed to coitus, coupled with preparatory concomitant or consecutive maltreatment.[7]

Note how he describes the behavior of a sexual act being fueled by the "maltreatment" of another human. You can also see that he believes the amount of discomfort felt by the victim is a direct factor in the degree of sexual gratification.

The term *sadism* originally described a behavior, not a psychological disorder. Subsequently, the psychiatric community attached the classification of *paresthesia* (an abnormal or perverse sexual feeling) to it. In 1980, the American Psychiatric Association changed the classification of sadism from a paresthesia to a *paraphilia* (a recurring sexual fantasy or behavior that involves unusual and especially socially unacceptable sexual practices), which is how it is still classified.[8]

The behavior associated with sadism has not changed since it was first defined. What has changed is the American Psychiatric Association's classification and diagnostic criteria for sadism and our view of what is healthy and unhealthy sadism. Today, if the sadism is consensual and not harmful to the person or to others, the association does not consider it to be a paraphilia. It is only labeled a paraphilia when it is deemed unhealthy and causes the person significant distress, and then it is defined as a psychosexual disorder comprising thoughts, sexual fantasies, or acts with nonconsenting persons or objects involving pain or humiliation of oneself or another.[9] Even the American Psychiatric Association says you can consent to pain and suffering!

WHAT'S PAIN GOT TO DO WITH IT?

The acronym BDSM is relatively new when compared to behaviors it describes, which date back more than two millennia. Within the BDSM community, the term *sadism* has mutated into something it is not. While we do know the origin of the word and the context in which it was first used, the old definition has become bastardized. Someone once said to me, "I suppose you could argue that it is not sadistic to give someone something they somehow enjoy, but in our world, sadism tends to be more about who is delivering the pain, not about how it is received." There does not need to be, nor should there be, any modification to the term *sadism* other than adding the word *consensual*. If you do not fit the behavior, don't change the established definition of a word that describes the behavior to make it fit you. Don't say you're a Sadist; just say you are topping someone. While some may complain that they hate labels and definitions, the language we use is important for communication and general understanding.

> *Now, consider this idea: a masochist is a Sadist's worst enemy. I say this somewhat tongue in cheek to get people to think about what "painful" sensations are really like for a masochist.*

After considering the behaviors encompassed by consensual sadism, it is vital to perceive and interpret the intent of the individual creating the sensations as well as what the bottom actually experiences.

Pain is defined as an unpleasant sensation resulting from physical trauma, disease, or an emotional disorder, suffering, or distress. This suggests that the person who feels pain is not happy about it. For example, undergoing dental work is painful for most of us, though I am sure there are a few people out there who enjoy the sensation of dental work. Note how I changed the word *pain* to *sensation* in that example.

We feel sensations when our senses are stimulated. Thus, sensations are highly individual and idiosyncratic to each of us; they can be interpreted in many ways. Some sensations can be pleasurable while others can be unpleasant. We define pain as an unpleasant sensation; people go to great lengths—think of pain clinics—not to feel it. Pain hurts people.

Now, consider this idea: a masochist is a Sadist's worst enemy. I say this somewhat tongue in cheek to get people to think about what "painful" sensations are really like for a masochist. What the rest of us would identify as pain and perceive as negative, masochists interpret differently. To them, it's a pleasurable, positive experience; thus, it is not pain.

You see, masochists do feel and interpret some sensations as painful, as hurting. Pain is only pain when the person receiving it interprets it as a negative or unpleasant sensation or one that causes suffering. I may think I am causing someone pain because, well—damn—it sure looks like it would hurt me. But in reality, he enjoys the sensation and doesn't experience it as "bad" pain.

This brings to mind tattoo work. While speaking with my tattoo artist, he told me that often, when he tattoos someone, he has to stop and give them a break because it hurts them too much. This applies to all areas of the body that he has worked on. While getting work done on the base of my neck, I started to laugh because it tickled. It held up his work because I had to settle myself down and hold still. But he told me this is a very painful place to tattoo for some people.

I will interject a theory here. Some believe that pain and pleasure are on the same continuum of sensation as interpreted by the mind. For example, a sensation like having your feet caned is extremely painful to some. For a masochist, it can feel pleasurable at first, but if continued long enough or delivered hard enough, the stimulus will eventually become painful. The masochist could become sexually aroused from a caning during the pleasurable stage, but would feel pain from the same activity further down the road.

Sadism is often misunderstood by our own BDSM community as a self-centered "dark" endeavor. Some wonder how a Sadist could possibly find a willing partner who submits to painful activities they don't enjoy. This always makes me chuckle. I am a known Sadist and I have no problem getting people to let me do unpleasant stuff to them. I always reveal what I am up front by giving partners my definition of sadism—I want to make them feel unpleasant sensations from which I will get sexual gratification when they dislike what I do—and they still want to give it a go. Sadism becomes abuse when the bottom no longer consents to the pain or when the bottom's needs are not met.

SADISM AND CONSENT

Often the consensual Sadists within the kink community use the term *consensual non-consensuality* or CNC (also referred to as *consensual nonconsent*) to describe certain scenes. Our community has been discussing this controversial practice for many years. If there is ever a dull moment in a discussion group or an online list, this is one issue—along with safewords and extreme scenes—that is guaranteed to liven things up.

I recall reading that CNC was a very heated topic of discussion at the National Leather Association's fifth conference in October 1990. In a postpanel interview conducted by Carol

Queen, the late Tony DeBlase was quoted concerning CNC: "A bottom may set parameters and say, 'Now, given those parameters, don't pay any attention to what I say after this.' We've gotten so much into negotiations and safewords that there are people who can't even conceive scening without them. They confuse consensual non-consensuality scenes with entirely non-consensual ones—which they aren't."

CNC remains no less controversial today. There are some who feel it is in direct violation of the seemingly universal BDSM guideline known as safe, sane, and consensual (SSC). When the phrase "risk-aware consensual kink" (RACK) was coined, it seemed to open a little more tolerance for CNC, simply because people were more willing to admit that there is some risk to many of our practices. But I have a personal issue with grouping sadism and "kink" together. Sorry, but equating the word "kink" to sadism is like comparing a bunny-fur flogger to a barbed-wire flogger. We all use catchphrases to simplify our conversations, often using our local group's shorthand. However, once we start to travel or speak outside our own leather community, we find that interpretations vary widely.

Those who practice CNC generally do not use safewords, and this causes a portion of the community to promptly condemn the practice. Many BDSM practitioners hold the opinion that a bottom should never give up the right to use a safeword under any circumstances. Yet an opposing segment of the leather/fetish community chooses not to use safewords for various reasons. Some are bottoms who feel they cannot go as far in a scene as they wish to if they have a safeword. Perhaps an even more motivating factor is fear of the unknown. Some get off on fear; not everyone gets off on knowing exactly what is going to happen to them.

To consent is "to give assent or approval."[10] To be nonconsensual is to disagree with what is proposed by another. So, by logical sequence, CNC in SM would be an agreement to not necessarily be in agreement with the actions that are forthcoming. Some consensual slaves and other bottoms receive a great deal of satisfaction through unconditionally submitting to the will of another. It is through the process of giving total control to another that they achieve deep submission, leading to spiritual well-being. It takes great strength and overwhelming trust to place total control in the hands of a Sadist, Top or Dominant. This exchange of power should never be granted thoughtlessly. Immense self-discipline, sterling character, and responsibility are required of the Top not to abuse such power once it has been given. However, I do not believe that an individual who has consented to forgoing the use of a safeword has given up their human right to stop an unsafe scene.

As Sadists, we know bottoms are getting something from letting us hurt them. In the moment, those who subject themselves to Sadists are in real pain and would rather be someplace else. That does not mean they don't later masturbate to the memory of the encounter. It could be that it is an act of service. In such cases, the individual will endure pain because they take pleasure in knowing they make the Sadist happy. It can also be an act of love, as is the case for my wife. There are times when I have sex with my wife when she is emotionally distraught and feeling "real" pain. As a consensual Sadist, it makes me happy to know that the encounter was good, at some point, for my wife. Yes, she was really hurting and hating me in the moment, which makes me come, but she is happy after it is over. I do not think anyone would consent to a Sadist if they got nothing from it.

Some feel that there are only sexual masochists in the BDSM community, but there are people who want to feel pain for the sake of feeling pain. They have a need to be beat to catharsis. They want to cry and purge by suffering in order to learn about themselves. I have done scenes with my wife simply for the sake of her suffering pain. She was not interested in feeling anything pleasurable in the moment. She wanted to feel catharsis. Can I get off sexually by this? Hell, yeah! However, in scenes like this, I am in a different role—more like a spiritual guide or facilitator for her journey.

When it comes to topping, you may hear additional descriptors attached to the word, such as "service Top" and "sensual Top." One term that really demonstrates a gross misunderstanding of sadism is "sensual Sadist." I mean, really? People use this term to explain that they are giving the bottom sensual sensations that the bottom likes to have done to them. There is nothing in it about pain, suffering, or dislike. This is not sadism.

So how far does a Sadist need to go to obtain sexual satisfaction? A Sadist only needs to go to the point where the bottom no longer enjoys what is taking place. This can happen in a matter of minutes or take as long as a few hours. I guess, by default, someone uses his safeword when he no longer enjoys what's happening. But certainly one could be in an unhappy state *before* using the safeword. So, in any scene where I am being a Sadist and a bottom calls a safeword, I am happy. Also, if I end the scene, it is because I feel they have gone far enough and should not be pushed further; again, I am happy. Have I ever been unhappy because I did not think a partner functioned well? Never. On the other hand, I have been unhappy with what a few partners did with what they were given. My sexual satisfaction does not have to end with penetration or with me having an orgasm.

AFTERCARE/AFTERMATH

The aftermath of sadism must be taken into account when looking at healthy, consensual sadism. I say *aftermath* because of the way my wife looks just after I've had sex with her. There she lies, on the floor, covered in sweat, tears, blood, and snot, looking as if she just went to hell and back. So, yeah, *aftermath* is a good term, I think. What I will talk about is what goes through my head and heart after taking her into the abyss. The consensual Sadist needs as much, if not more, aftercare than the bottom. This is simply because we are doing things to people that they don't like.

Certainly there can be scenes involving acts of consensual nonconsent which, if taken alone, can appear to be nonabusive. But what happens after the scene is just as important, if not more so. If I leave my wife in a pool of blood, sweat, and tears after a consensual rape scene and *never* tend to her afterward, this would be abusive. We must look out for the physical and emotional well-being of the bottom after the scene ends. If the bottom's needs are realistic and within reason and they are not met, it is abusive.

Taking everything into account, there really is no good reason for us to distance ourselves from our roots. What the Marquis de Sade wrote about were primarily nonconsensual acts. These are not the roots that I am talking about. I am talking about pure, hot, sexually charged consensual sadism, where your partner agrees to feel pain because it gets you off.

The psychological effects that consensual Sadists have on the bottoms they play with can be devastating if there are misunderstandings. Suppose a bottom has done scenes only with tops who inflicted sensations that the bottom liked, and those tops called themselves Sadists. Then, if a consensual Sadist were to create unpleasant sensations for the bottom—because that is what a consensual Sadist does—the inexperienced and poorly educated bottom freaks out. This does not do the consensual Sadist any good either, having a bottom react poorly. Who knows where it could go from there.

People do recruit into the lifestyle. We bring in new people fresh out of their closets and make them feel comfortable with words like *play* and *toys*. Acronyms like SSC and RACK make newbies feel safe from harm, I guess. I take exception to the words *play* and *toys*. At one time what we did was called "working a boy over." What we used were tools, not toys.

So here we have the preprogrammed recruit, the "SSC sadistic Top," using "toys" in a "play" session at a public BDSM event. She happens to look over and see what I would call a real consensual Sadist, whose bottom does not look as if he is enjoying what is being done to him. The bottom is even saying, "No, stop!" Holy bat droppings, Batman!!! The SSC sadistic Top thinks, That must be nonconsensual and unsafe. Get a

Dungeon Monitor quick—that scene must be stopped. Do you see how not giving the full picture of sadism can be harmful to our community? We must learn to communicate our needs better as Sadists, Dominants, or Tops. Bottoms, if a person says she is a Sadist, ask her what that means. It's a necessary conversation, where people can express their personal definitions and desires and establish a clearer understanding. Then, if all goes well, you can get down to some hot sadistic sex.

Endnotes

1. Ovid (43 BC–AD 17), *The Art of Love*, quoted in *Sexual Life in Ancient Rome*, by Otto Kiefer (Taylor & Francis, 1956), 239.
2. Richard Freiherr von Krafft-Ebing, *Psychopathia Sexualis* (Stuttgart, Germany: Verlag Von Ferdinand Enke, 1886), 109.
3. In addition, subsequent behavioral descriptors of sadism do not include behavior toward animals.
4. Marquis de Sade, *The 120 Days of Sodom and Other Writings* (New York: Grove Press, 1987), 642.
5. Marquis de Sade, 642.
6. Marquis de Sade, *Justine, The Complete Marquis de Sade, Volume 1*, John S. Yankowski, trans. (Los Angeles: Holloway House Publishing, 2005), 65.
7. Krafft-Ebing, 53.
8. This general definition of paraphilia is from *Merriam-Webster's Collegiate Dictionary*, 11th ed. Psychiatric definition: "The essential features of a Paraphilia are recurrent, intense sexually arousing fantasies, sexual urges or behaviors generally involving (1) nonhuman objects, (2) the suffering or humiliation of oneself or one's partner, or (3) children or other nonconsenting persons that occur over a period of at least 6 months." *The Diagnostic and Statistical Manual of Mental Disorders* (DSM-IV-TR), American Psychiatric Association (Arlington, VA: American Psychiatric Publishing, 2000), 573.
9. The language of the DSM-IV-TR reads: "The diagnosis is made if the behavior [see previous note], sexual urges, or fantasies cause clinically significant distress or impairment in social, occupational, or other important areas of functioning." American Psychiatric Association, 573.
10. *Merriam-Webster's Collegiate Dictionary*, 11th ed.

CHAPTER 17

AGE ROLE PLAY
IGNACIO RIVERA, AKA PAPÍ COXXX

Has anyone ever told you not to do something and you thought to yourself, Why can't I do it? Or, If I did it, would it hurt anybody? You find yourself thinking of ways to get your mind off the thing you're not supposed to do, but you can't. The restriction itself propels you to want to do it. It's exciting, alluring. For some people, that's what it feels like to do age role play, both sexual and nonsexual: it's taboo. For others, it's rooted in pure desire. It just gets you downright hot. Still others engage in age play to explore a specific dynamic with a partner or partners. Age play offers people the opportunity to explore a wonderful childhood memory or a time when their lives were simpler and without responsibility. They can sexualize a forbidden intergenerational relationship or indulge in a wide variety of Dominant/submissive power dynamics.

Fantasy role play is when two or more consenting adults engage in intentional erotic or power-dynamic-driven interactions. Age play is a specific form of fantasy role play where a partner embodies a person of a different age than their actual chronological age. Age-play characters run the gamut from diapered babies and little girls to rowdy teenagers and dirty old men. For some people, age play is a chance to return to a younger age and engage with other adults who are role-playing their peers: think Boy Scouts roughhousing together. Other folks want to be youths or children and interact with partners who take on an adult role: the troublemaking student in detention under the watchful eye of a stern teacher, or an infant who gets to be pampered and loved by a wonderful nanny; the "adult" in these scenarios almost always has some power over the "kid." Some people enjoy playing persons older than themselves to take on a role of authority or embody a parental figure. Others employ age play to engage in scenarios where their partners play a relative (some call this "familial age play" or "incest play"): for example, a seven-year-old who loves to color with her dad or two adolescent brothers who explore their bodies together.

Age play can be quite taboo, not only in society at large, but also among kinky people. After all, adults are not *supposed* to act like children, and once an erotic interaction is introduced, things get even dicier. Some people automatically associate age play with pedophilia, child sexual abuse, and sex offenders. Before we go any further, I must be very clear. Age play is exactly what the name indicates—*play*. If you have a desire to do age play, it does not mean you condone coercion, violence, or abuse (sexual or nonsexual) directed at *actual* children by *actual* adults. Age play is fantasy between consenting adults.

> Age play is edge play for me. It takes me to wonderfully enlightening places as well as deep, dark ones.

Whatever age I choose to play, a scene can have very different outcomes, but the main thread in age play for me is sex. It can involve an intricacy of domination, incest, rape, and sometimes torture. Age play is edge play for me. It takes me to wonderfully enlightening places as well as deep, dark ones. I allow myself to balance and sometimes fall off the edges—that's what makes it hot for me. There are people who do nonsexual age play, but this chapter focuses on age play with an erotic component.

There are many ways to figure out what age play may look like for you. I'm a visual person, so creating lists helps me collect and organize my thoughts, clarify my vision for the scene, and figure out logistics. I like to think of it as working in your own laboratory. In the laboratory, you can create any concoction of age play you desire. Think of the choices as chemicals. Making a choice about what you want today does not mean you can't switch, alter, reconfigure, or change your mind about the whole idea of what age play looks like to you. Don't worry, you are entitled to change your formula. You are the evil scientist of your desires.

> # THE LABORATORY CHECKLIST
>
> Role
> Age
> Gender
> Sexual orientation
> Power dynamic
> Relationship and connection
> Private or public
> Frequency
> Props, costumes, scene elements

SQUARE ONE

If you've been curious about age play or about how to spice it up with some hot sex, it's good to step back and start at square one: what was the fantasy or the initial thought? One of the most difficult tasks is sifting through our fantasies and figuring out what we want to make "reality." Reality in this context is creating the scenario that mirrors what has been living in your brain—making tangible the thing that gets you off. Sometimes we figure out that the fantasy we've had for years lives best as only a fantasy. There is nothing wrong with that. Some fantasies we birth and others we carry. We can play with them in our minds or in real life—the choice is yours. I took the plunge and decided once and for all that the fantasy I'd been jerking off to for 10 years was worth acting out. Taking that plunge for you may mean taking baby steps.

A conversation about the topic of erotic age play is a good

place to begin with a partner. The goal is to figure out if all parties are at least interested and are not repulsed or triggered by the idea. You can bring up a blog you read or pop a porn scene featuring some kind of age play in the DVD player. Or you can just straight-out ask your partner how age play sounds to them. Gauge your partner's reaction. Notice your reaction. If all feels right at the moment, move forward. Talk about what turns you on about an age play scenario. Describe how you see yourself in the scenario and why you want to be in it. Answering the "why" is important in that it propels you to create intent and allows the other players to understand their role if they chose to agree to it. For some, this method of asking yourself who and why is essential; for others, the need just is—there is no need to analyze the desire. Some are drawn to age play but are not sure where to start.

Take it slow at first. Try a 15-minute session rather than a two-hour session. Check in with each other afterward. Did it feel good? Did it feel weird? Are you willing to try it again or put it back in your brain vault? Weather you never delve into that fantasy again or you move forward with it, it's totally okay. You took the plunge, landed on your feet, and now you know. Unfortunately, some of us may not land so gracefully. There is nothing wrong with you. Our journeys take us to different destinations.

CHOOSING YOUR AGE

When you fantasize about age play, what age are you? Does it shift? Is it always the same? Age play can be regressive or progressive. The more common type of age play involves at least one partner regressing in age; progressing to an older age is less common. I have been a newborn and I've been 80 years old.

Regressing to a younger age can be about a longing to relive or recreate childhood experiences. Are you a baby? All babies are preverbal, helpless, and dependent on a parent or caregiver for everything. Are you a good baby or a naughty one? Maybe you're a kid. Kids can talk and do some things for themselves, but they are still dependent on adults; they often express their thoughts without worrying about what people think. Kids have unique personalities: they can be shy, tantrum-throwing, naive, eager to please, or bratty. Perhaps you'd like to be a teenager, somewhat independent yet still not a grown-up. Are you curious about sex, rebellious, a teacher's pet? Think about what you want to get out of this role play and what age range is most appealing to you.

In age progression, you can progress to as little as a few years older than your actual age or all the way up to senior status. I suspect that age progression, also known as elder play or geriatric play, is not considered as fantastical as regressing to your youth. The age process creates fear in most people and may limit how your play is acted out or evolves. Age progression may be too close to the reality of growing up, growing old, or being ill. Regression eliminates impending reality, sparks memory, and allows room for mistakes, or it is just plain fun. I would argue, though, that elder play can be just as naughty, taboo, and creative as a youthful tryst. Progressive age play can be anything from a candy striper in a nursing home blowing an elderly gentleman to Grandpa making his granddaughter sit on his lap as he feels under her dress, or—my personal favorite—a senior patient getting a special sponge bath from the hot young nurse.

GENDER AND SEXUAL ORIENTATION

So, you are thinking that if you identify as a female, your role-play alter egos have to be female, too? Absolutely not. Do you want to be a little girl, an adult male, a gender-transitioning youth, a gender-nonconforming person, or an androgynous teen? Your physical body does not have to match the gender you want to role-play. You can have a penis and be a woman, have breasts and be a boy—you decide. I identify as a trans genderqueer person. In my play, I have been a seven-year-old girl seductress, a 20-year-old sexually assaultive jock, a dirty old man who is 80, a 30-year-old incestuous Daddi, and a feminine, sexually inappropriate boy who is 10.

The same goes for sexual orientation or behavior. You may have been born male and identify as such but in play you could be a lesbian or simply a woman who gets fucked by other women. You can also be a little girl who likes little boys, a teenage boy coming of age with other teenage boys, or a dirty mother who fucks her son and daughter. Remember, this is play and you and your partners can navigate it anyway you want. You can be queer, lesbian, heterosexual, bisexual, gay, asexual, fluid, or pansexual.

POWER DYNAMIC

It doesn't matter how old you are in the role play—you can still decide whether you are a top, bottom, or switch in the scenario. For example, my seven-year-old girl seductress waited until Daddy was asleep, then crawled into bed with him and sucked him off. When he realized what was happening and wanted to stop it, I threatened to tell. Age does not dictate the power you have in your role play. Your great-uncle on his deathbed could be the top in your role play scenario. He can determine that when he passes on, you get all of his inheritance—but for a detailed sexual price. You could have a student who holds all the cards when she reveals to you she has sexually incriminating evidence of your raunchy sex life. She'll keep her mouth shut for a passing grade and a good fuck. The bad guys can be the tops in a child abduction, rape, and torture scenario. The babysitter can be the top when she spanks the youngsters she's babysitting for wetting the bed. It's all up to you. Have fun with it.

RELATIONSHIP AND CONNECTION

What connection do the players have? Do you know each other, live together, or have you never met each other? There are many exciting ways to relate to one another in age play; with each type of connection, you can explore trust, love, friendship, fear, or resiliency. Perhaps you are members of the same family: parents, grandparents, guardians, uncles, aunts, children, siblings, nieces and nephews. There are many scenes involving young people and adult authority figures such as teachers, tutors, priests, babysitters, neighbors, school counselors, coaches, ballet instructors. Less well known adult authority figures include doctor, camp counselor, corner store clerk, postal worker, and bus driver. A stranger might be part of your age play—perhaps a hitchhiker, a kidnapper, or the person passing you on the street. Whether the connection you create is a brief encounter with the bus driver or an ongoing relationship with your brother, each connection can spark an array of creative scenarios to explore.

PUBLIC/PRIVATE

Where will you set the stage for your encounter? Will your interactions take place at home, at a public kink event, or among the general public? If you are dipping your toes into the pool of age play, a more private location is suggested. Private play is more intimate: you don't have to factor in uncontrolled input from the outside world, so it can feel safer. At a kink party or conference, there may be special activities or space reserved for regressive age players (often called "kidz" or "littles"). In these kinky spaces, you can meet and interact with other age players, feel acknowledged as your alter ego, play, compare notes, etc.

FREQUENCY

Is this something you're curious about and you'd like to try once? Do you want to do it on occasion to spice up your sex life? Or is it play that you want to develop and do on a regular basis? Do you want to incorporate age play into your 24/7 D/s dynamic? You don't have to know the answers right away; these are lifestyle options to consider. Play can happen once or sporadically. A scenario can incorporate the same characters or different ones. Scenarios don't necessarily have to mature. And long-term investment in the role play is not essential. I have done one-time scenes as well as created continuing characters who reappear again and again. I have been developing one of my little personas for years. Creating a continuing character has helped me tap into the psyche of the character and develop her more fully: she has a name, a birth date, a family history, and memories. I have invested time, money, and emotions in her, and this makes for a richer, more complex experience when I embody her in a scene. She has grown and changed over the years, and so have I.

PROPS, COSTUMES, SCENE ELEMENTS

When it comes to role playing, our imaginations can take us to faraway, wonderful places. Props and costumes can help propel the imagination, but keep in mind that you don't need to spend a lot of money to get into the perfect head space. Shopping at secondhand stores or getting hand-me-downs from friends are a great way to obtain a variety of clothes and props to play with. A coloring book, a box of cereal, Grandpa's cane, Daddy's pipe, Mama's purse, diapers, or a stuffed animal are all exciting elements you can add to your play. These items allow us to fall deeper into our roles—make us connect to what our alter egos like, do, use, or need. I have a second pair of glasses I call my "girl" glasses. When those glasses rest on my face, I am transformed. Do you fantasize about sucking on a pacifier? Does a lollipop bring out your inner toddler? Think about items that connect you to your character, embrace them, and have some fun.

NEGOTIATION

In the process of making your own laboratory list, think about what your particular role means to you and work on verbalizing it to your play partners. Simply saying that you are interested in embodying a "dirty older brother" is not enough. Different roles, especially familial ones, can be interpreted in different ways and will often reflect your background, race, culture, ethnicity, or religion. You want to make sure that you and your role-paying partners are on the same page. If not, the scene may go in the wrong direction or can even be triggering. The same goes for a player who asks her partner to play a specific character. You can say you want a daddy, but what does Daddy mean to you? Is he stern and punishing, gentle and caring, or something else altogether? Finding clarity about characters can be difficult—we must dig deep, examine, and name what turns us on. The outcome of this internal work can be rewarding.

There are various precautions you and your partner(s) should also discuss when negotiating. You have to take proactive as well as possibly reactive measures. If there's anything the BDSM scene prepares you for, it is that anything can happen. I think that's the sheer beauty of it. When you role-play, you imagine and create new worlds, new temporary realities, and those realities can be both good and bad.

Just as a top asks a bottom about past injuries in order to assess areas of the body to avoid hitting, the players in age play should talk about past emotional traumas and triggers. For example, I had a fuck buddy who role-played a teenager who was raped by her neighbor, played by me. When negotiating the terms of our play, she revealed that she was once assaulted and during the assault she was choked. She told me that anything around her neck would trigger her, so we agreed that choking or using a collar was a no-no. Another play partner let me know that I should not address her as "honey." She had been sexually harassed and the perpetrator consistently used that endearment to minimize her.

> Age play can be healing and therapeutic for some people, but it is not the same as therapy.

Knowing people's individual triggers helps you avoid pushing the wrong buttons in a scene; however, you cannot always prepare for what might come up. During age play, people can regress to a much younger age that can bring up intense primal or instinctual feelings. It can put both top and bottom in a very delicate head space, so you must keep that in mind. Even when you plan ahead, all scenes have the potential to go south. Be open to that. Accept it. Knowing this can allow you to be more receptive and as ready as you can be to react to a situation you did not plan on.

Age play can be a highly emotional and challenging journey for survivors and their partners, for those who love us and those who play with us. Age play can be healing and therapeutic for some people, but it is not the same as therapy; this is especially important to note for survivors of childhood incest, sexual abuse, or trauma. Age play, accompanied by therapy, the support of friends, and artistic outlets, has been extremely healing for me. This will not be the case for all survivors. We find what healing paths work best for us.

When you combine age play with incest play—scenarios like Daddy/girl, Mommy/boy, Sister/brother, Uncle/nephew—it can take your play to a whole new level. It can be based in nurturing, caregiving, letting go, emotional exploration, trust, tapping into your inner child, reliving, and more. Think about some of your core truths and you may discover some of your core fantasies. Is it to feel the undeniable love of a mother? The sexual taboo of incest? Mix in consensual coercion, fear and terror, rape and abuse fantasies, and you've got all the ingredients for a very intense scene. This kind of age play is not for everyone. It can be exciting yet explosive. Exploring taboo subjects can open up emotional floodgates. So it's key to negotiate, renegotiate, and check in. Checking in directly after a scene can be enough for some, but others may need hourly check-ins, maybe a check-in days later. This type of play may bring to the surface sadness, anger, fear and hatred—in yourself and your partner. Navigating the root of the feeling and dealing with it appropriately can be a challenge, but it is an important part of understanding the responsibilities of playing on the edge. We have a responsibility to ourselves and those we play with. This is why honest, clear communication and negotiation is key.

One thing we can plan for is aftercare: what takes place

after a session. It's the attention you give one another emotionally and physically. Aftercare is for both tops and bottom. Like other BDSM activities, age play can drain us, especially emotionally. Aftercare is a wonderful way to be taken care of, revitalize, and come back to embodying *you* again. Aftercare looks different for many people. It can be minimal, or as detailed as the players want it to be. I know people who just want a cup of water and to be left alone for a while. Others need constant touch and affirmation. Still others want no verbal communication, just to be held tight. Whatever your aftercare needs, remember to discuss beforehand.

I've laid out some tools based on personal experience, conversations, and writings on the subject that I hope will help you and your partner(s) understand and navigate age role play. Experimenting with age play can be scary but it can also be extremely fulfilling. Sexual age play is vast, dirty, and desired by many. Take time to figure out what turns you on about it. Sit with it. Fantasize about it. Jerk off or touch yourself to the possibilities of it. Decide whether you want to take your desires from fantasy to reality. Communicate openly and as honestly as possible with your fuck buddies, lovers, play partners, or spouses. Play to your heart's content. Listen to your inner voice and concoct all the sexual age play you desire.

CHAPTER 18

DIGGING IN THE DIRT: THE LURE OF TABOO ROLE PLAY

MOLLENA WILLIAMS

Author's Note: I recommend that you read Chapter 11, Stop, Drop, and Role! Erotic Role Playing, before reading this essay. It will help provide context. Okay—let's rock.

Naughty is nice. Bad is good. Evil is better. Violence is love and fantasy is a secret passageway into a reality gone deliciously, dangerously, erotically haywire.

You with me? Good. It only gets darker from here.

One of the aspects of role play that I love is taking responsibility for abdicating responsibility. How is this paradox possible? By enacting a scenario where you take or relinquish control, you inhabit a sexually charged world of endless possibility. By negotiating your scenario including your limits and boundaries, and mapping out expectations and outcomes, you create a matrix into which you can insert your dreams, fantasies, and darkest desires. This liberates the role players, giving them the freedom to explore some of humanity's darkest impulses, and to explore them without the limiting trappings of guilt, apprehension, and fear. Sound intriguing? Want to jump right into that hot-and-heavy rape fantasy? Ease back there, my friend. There is a lot to dig up, uncover, and sift through before you jump into the deep end.

Uncovering the roots of your desires can truly assist in your explorations, especially if you are experiencing guilt around wanting to ravage—or be ravaged by—another human. It is not easy to get to the point of being comfortable even thinking about some of the darker fantasies that many people entertain in the recesses of their hearts. I know that, for me, it was a multistage process and remains an ongoing one.

One of the earliest sexual memories I have is the fantasy of being overpowered, ravaged, taken against my will, and forced to submit to a power I cannot resist. Every captured-princess tale whispered to me of secrets behind the gauzy veils and pointed hats. The creaking wire bookstands in the supermarket were packed with racks of romance novels. The covers of these pulp fictions depicted heaving-bosomed and wild-eyed women resisting, pushing, straining against broad-shouldered, thickly muscled men who smiled arrogantly, seemingly impervious to the willowy resistance of the heroine. One of my favorite *Star Trek* episodes, "Space Seed," included a rather evocative scene in which the villain, Kahn Noonian Singh (played with smoldering sensuality by a young

Ricardo Montalban), seduced, overpowered, and dominated a crewmember of the Enterprise into crawling, pleading, abject submission. I looked to those fantasies, told over and over in different forms and narratives, as confirming my desire to be overpowered, to be ravaged. Until reality hit me and I became convinced that my desires, my fantasies, were wrong. Very fucking wrong.

As a child, watching the miniseries *Roots* was a major event for me, and everyone I knew watched it. It was especially gripping, as a black kid, to see the story of people who looked like me, people with a similar ancestral history, unfolding in epic glory night after night. I was swept away in surges of emotion: pride at their bravery in the face of oppression, rage at the evils of enforced slavery, fear at the pain and suffering depicted, rather graphically, in the story. But the biggest conflict for me came up in the scene where a white man forcibly rapes a black female slave. This was not the sexy ravishment of those Harlequin Romance novels. This was not a whispered fairy tale, where allegory and wistful gasps and sighs gave only hints of secret lust. This was brutal violence, horrible and horrifying, and I couldn't understand how something that looked so much like my fantasies left me sick and terrified. And fascinated.

Unable to make sense of this dichotomy, I internalized the idea that there was something profoundly wrong with me, that I carried a secret I could never, ever share. I knew that there had to be a difference between the fantasies I had and the reality depicted in this scene of brutal violence, but—they *looked* the same. What *was* the difference?

The deeper and darker a secret feels, the more likely it's a common one. When I became old enough to take control of my own fantasies and let go of my initial fear of being "sick" for having these thoughts, I discovered that not only was I not alone, but these fantasies were common. My first boyfriend and I played with resistance in our sex: "You want it, I got it, I ain't givin' it to ya without a fight!" Sometimes he would let me overpower him, and I would exert my own power, with much delight. And sometimes I would find myself overpowered, taken, and ravaged to my heart's content. This was still not something I felt I could share with anyone but him, but it was a delicious secret that we shared and we thoroughly enjoyed its transgressive energy.

These early explorations might never have blossomed into a deeper, darker journey save for a brief incandescent affair I had in my mid-twenties. Previously, any rough sex I'd had was playful, contextualized, and something both parties had to agree to for any play to begin.

Then I encountered someone who did *not* ask, did *not* negotiate, took what he wanted with no preamble. And I found that…irresistible.

It was a revelation to have an encounter with a man who was effortlessly dominant, sexually aggressive, and able to read me so well that even my stunned responses and token resistance did not slow his roll. Previously, any sexual aggression I'd absorbed had taken place after explicit communication. This was not so clear. He pushed, I acquiesced. He pushed harder, I retreated. He demanded, I crumbled. He took what he wanted, I gave it up with a delicate blend of relief, fear, and confused arousal. Here was exactly what I had secretly craved: someone who knew, just knew, my deep, dark secret who took one look at me and reached inside to that dark place and exploited it for his own pleasure. And ultimately for mine.

> *Fantasizing about acts that are manifestations of nonconsensual encounters is one thing. Deciding to consciously explore them is another.*

As I unpacked this experience and started sharing it with trusted friends, no one chastised me for my fantasy. Friends nodded, a gleam in their eyes, asked for details, wanted to know what happened next. And next. I realized I wasn't on the fringe. Not by a long shot. And I wanted more.

But getting more presented a substantial challenge.

Fantasizing about acts that are manifestations of nonconsensual encounters is one thing. Deciding to consciously explore them is another. I think we can all agree that the violence of rape and sexual assault, the violence of bigotry and racism, the horror of sexual abuse, the crime and horror of incest, are not acceptable. They are inexcusable, criminal acts of violence.

So how can it be that so many of us have fantasies along these lines? How can it be that, in one breath, I can condemn the rapist and yet fantasize about being ravaged and raped?

INTENT AND CONSENT

There are two fundamental concepts here: consent and intent.

The *intent* of those participating in taboo role play is not to harm others. Their intent may vary. It can be a reclamation, a re-creation, an exploration—but it is *never* a decimation, an obliteration of the humanity of the people involved. Intent is all-important when diving into these dark waters.

Consent is also pivotal. Inasmuch as a person who engages in a fantasy about being used and degraded by a terrifying sexual predator has consented to the scenario being manifested, the acts are elevated above criminality. Rape, incest, abuse based on race, gender, sexual preference, or physical ability are not acceptable—*unless they are*. Once these taboos are brought to light as a forbidden fruit that the participants willingly, and with open eyes, choose to ingest, the game is entirely different. It can be transmuted, with negotiation and consent, to a profound exploration of the darkness within us all. It can be everything from light and fun to darkly cathartic.

But you must enter into this maze with a grounded sense of yourself, your motives, and your desires, and an awareness of the inherent and hidden risks.

Let me be very clear. I am in no way condoning any behavior that is nonconsensually perpetrated upon another person as a means of physical and emotional violence. Rather, I am saying that those who desire to explore these fantasies in the context of a consensual, self-aware, intentional exploration of personal desires ought not be reflexively pathologized. I believe that these fantasies can be deeply empowering, and we should give ourselves permission to dig in this dirt.

It is vital to understand that consent must be granted by all involved parties when exploring scenarios that employ physical manifestations of violence and psychological shades of coercion. As someone who has been on the receiving end of sexual assault, I can tell you firsthand that there is a universe of difference between the dark seduction of a rape-play fantasy and fighting off a would-be attacker or being taken advantage of via emotional pressure or coercion. Consent and choice are what sets this type of play apart from abuse and assault. I choose the time, the place and the partners with whom I play in this realm. I make the decision with a clear-eyed and sober mind-set. I negotiate and I check in. I know my partners will be with me before, throughout, and in the aftermath of our shared experience. And I know that they care for me. The sexual abuser or rapist is not in the business of negotiation and thoughtful, caring planning. Your fantasy and desire is not their[1] concern.

Playing in the realm of *consensual nonconsent* may blur the lines of default "No means no!" language. But remember, *all involved parties must give consent to and accept responsibility for the risks associated with these boundary-pushing scenes*. Everyone assumes a risk. Being aware of and prepared for these risks is pivotal. Maintaining boundaries is not something to be compromised.

WHY GO THERE?

Taboo role play is heavy stuff, for sure. So why go there? Why dabble in behavior that tips on the edge of consent? There are as many reasons as there are people who choose to walk these dark paths. Some people are simply sexually curious—dark fantasies arouse their inquisitiveness, so they go for it. Others have demons they wish to exorcise, fears that are rooted in a very real situation that they seek to recast and over which they seek to gain control. This type of role play is a means by which they might access that past. Still others are specifically aroused by the forbidden nature of it. The edgier and riskier the game, the more desirable it is to play.

I have spoken to thousands of people in the kink/leather/BDSM community, and thousands who are not involved with this subculture, about their private sexual fantasies. What I find striking is that among those who are not actively leading a lifestyle that openly embraces kink, there is *less* stratification and judgment about the content of forbidden fantasies.

> *Many publicly eschew edge play, as it is called, and make an effort to demystify kink by downplaying the risks and the danger.*

Perverts often have a great deal invested, egowise, in codifying and justifying their kinks and fetishes. Many publicly eschew *edge play*, as it is called, and make an effort to demystify kink by downplaying the risks and the danger. Nonkink-identified people tend to have a "kinky is kinky" approach, which paradoxically gives them an initial advantage in processing taboo desires. When I came out to my nonkinky friends as submissive and confided that I was struggling with having fantasies that included scenes mirroring historical abuses, their reaction was generally "Okay, well that's pretty kinky!" Whereas revealing the same desires within BDSM communities earned me widespread ostracism, questioning of my "blackness," insinuations that I was mentally ill, threats against me and any potential partners "caught doing that fucked-up shit," and all manner of ridicule. Not all kinks are created equal.

One doesn't have to look far to find kinky people playing out the fantasy of the innocent schoolgirl/schoolboy over the knee of a stern disciplinarian. But darken the sexuality of it, add the sheen of sexual exploitation, coercion, or force, and the level of discomfort spikes. Reconciling something as horrific as the sexual abuse of children with the fantasy of playing that scene is a razor-edge dance. Many of our fantasies are rooted in real nightmares, fueled by the energy of real demons. But does this mean we ought to cut ourselves off from them, and in so doing, alienate ourselves from a base but valid aspect of our psyche? Does it mean we wish to *actually* abuse the innocent in a nonconsensual way? Does having a rape fantasy mean you desire to be beaten and sexually assaulted by a violent predator?

Most likely, the answer is no. But it is a *human* thing to desire to explore that destruction, that entropy, and there are safer ways to explore it. Just as we might watch a slasher flick to get that adrenaline rush of terror, we can put ourselves, for a little while, into a situation that feels very risky, that mimics that sickening rush of fear, so as to embrace the shadow of that horror.

SELF-EXPLORATION

To those who would explore these dark places, I first advise some really honest soul-searching. Where does this desire come from? Do you have a past hurt you would like to explore? Is it simply something that turns you on? Are you willing to deal with the possible aftermath: potential "buyer's remorse" after engaging in this play when you look back and second-guess your motives, and your partners'?

If you do have a past trauma, know that this play is not therapy. It may have a cathartic benefit, but it absolutely is neither a means to obtain mental health nor a substitute for frank discussions with a professional. I encourage survivors of abuse to explore their past with a kink-aware therapist or counselor prior to delving into this world. And I redouble that recommendation if you are contemplating engaging in edge play. A person who was raped at knifepoint and thinks that having someone they trust recreate the trauma will help them "get over it" is taking a risk—and putting their partner and their relationship at risk as well. Sure, it might all be peachy-keen and hugs and smiles afterward. But it might be profoundly triggering instead, and prove difficult for the surrogate perpetrator to recover from if the victim experiences difficulty in the scene's aftermath.

Everyone is at risk here. The risks to the bottom, the victim in this scenario, seem obvious. The potential for flashbacks or new traumas looms. But what about the aggressor, the perp? Are you sure, in the cold light of day, you won't look at the friend who did bad things to you and have flashbacks to the gravity of the scenario you brought to life? What happens if this doubt creates cracks in the foundation of your trust with them? If you are the wicked abuser, are you prepared to handle the feelings that might come up for you when you realize that you've unleashed a demon that deliberately pushed another human to the brink and possibly beyond? There is also the risk of transference. If a survivor of abuse replays the abuse in a role-playing scenario, there is a chance that unresolved issues may attach to the partner who has stepped into the role of the abuser, even if it is in the context of a consensual scene.

Knowing why all involved parties are up for this most dangerous game will help build the absolutely necessary trust and get everyone on the same page. Frank disclosure of personal histories, from all sides, is of vital importance. And self-care, including discussing your concerns and history with a health-care professional familiar with the practices of consensual BDSM, kink, and leathersex, is an essential step in processing those past traumas.

Each of us has our own darkness. What might seem a deeply disturbing scenario to one might be an average Thursday night for another. There are, however, some categories of dark role play that are generally regarded as edge play. These include, but aren't limited to, scenes of rape, domestic violence, hate crimes, and incest. The common thread in these scenarios is an effort by the aggressor to dehumanize, disempower, and control the victim for their own gratification. This is the taproot to the dark energy that can fuel these scenes. Power, forcefully taken, can be an intoxicant for the aggressor. And being stripped of one's power in a consensual role-play scene can also be titillating for the one being overpowered. A loss of control gives you permission to simply *be in that moment,* carried not by your own impulses and volition, but subject to the whims of the one who has coldly decided to make you fodder for their selfish desires. As troubling as these impulses may seem, when channeled through the stream of consensual play, they can be an outlet for impulses that deserve healthy release.

Rape and domestic abuse are never acceptable. There is no excuse, no defense, for emotional, physical, and psychological violence against another person. Then how does one justify these desires? It is simple to talk about consent, but there are those who assert that no one can ever *consent* to abuse. There is legal support for this position, as even consensual BDSM and kink behaviors are prosecutable offenses in most jurisdictions. So how can I say yes to saying "No!" but not meaning it? Am I not just mirroring the abuses around me by perpetrating these abuses in a fantasy that merely propagates a system designed to oppress and strip me of my humanity?

If my stated desires as an adult look like an abusive or dehumanizing interaction, and my partners and I make an informed decision to engage in it, it's all good, baby. Seriously. Acting out personal or historically wicked situations and/or abuses is my right. My sexual fulfillment is only as politicized as I permit it to be. I give no quarter to the juggernaut of political correctness when it aims for my libido, leaving behind a grease stain of shame and guilt.

I'm a black woman living in the USA. While there are people who experience a greater degree of socioeconomic and racial disadvantage, or who have more oppression pressure points to hit, there aren't many. So when I say I have struggled in the darkness of my own desires, trust that these were not easy to digest and overcome. My ancestors, my predecessors who fought for the rights of women and the rights of people of color were fighting for freedom, and I plan to respect their memory by exercising that freedom.

After struggling with the desire to be submissive *and a feminist*, wrestling with my secret cravings for rough, violent sexual encounters, denying my masochistic streak, vilifying my desire to be "owned" in the context of a consensual BDSM master/slave relationship *as the descendant of African slaves in the colonies*, I finally began to find peace when I realized I was not doing myself any favors by denying these desires. I need to live authentically. If there are things about my desires that shame me, and I succumb to that shame, I am not being true to myself. Rather than bury them, I have given myself permission to explore them, and I have found ways to plumb the depths of these desires with people who understand them and are willing to walk that dark path with me.

As I've mentioned previously, doing your homework is critical to mitigating risks in taboo role play. I say *mitigating* because nothing is 100 percent guaranteed. There *is* risk. That is part of the frisson of danger: we are walking that tightrope. There are many things to keep in mind when plotting these scenarios (for detailed information, I suggest reading my previous chapter, Stop, Drop, and Role! Erotic Role Playing) but the mind-set of the aggressor is key. In the case of a rape fantasy, for example, the motivation and the goal of the rapist needs to be absolutely clear.

I spoke to a fellow kink/BDSM educator about the preparatory work and personal exploration necessary to negotiate rape fantasies. Barak, in addition to having many years of experience as a health-care professional, has also worked as a nurse in a psychiatric crisis center. He and his wife, Sheba, founded Adventures in Sexuality (AIS), a group in the Midwest that focuses on education, outreach, and safety within the BDSM, kink, pansexual, and polyamorous communities. Since they conduct presentations centered around play that is edgy and pushes the edges of consent, and he has specific experience being the aggressor in scenes that play with themes of rape and consensual nonconsent, I asked Barak about the mind-set needed to successfully navigate these turbulent waters. This is his reply:

> It is tricky to approach playing with a rape fantasy, and the approach will vary depending on if it is a coercive "rough sex" scenario or a full-on consensual nonconsent scene. In the former, the eventual goal is mutual satisfaction. An example might be an overpoweringly coercive "date rape" fantasy where the "victim" is eventually, forcibly "seduced" to an erotic reaction and a sexualization of the power shift, even if it is not initially consensual. There can be a rather more playful approach to these scenes, without an overwhelmingly violent element.
>
> This becomes a different scene if the total stripping of power is the goal. Goals have to be clear in terms of the activity and the consequences. Rape is almost never about sex. It is about power and control.
>
> In the consensual nonconsent scenario, the participants agree to push past boundaries, regardless of the pleasure of the victim. There is a specific

disregard for the other person's satisfaction. In that case, the mind-set has to include objectification. Removing power and control, removing part of what makes them sentient, makes them an object upon which you feed. Dehumanizing them, reducing them to "food." Food for power, food for lust. As the one taking that power in that way, you can't have concern for your victim's feelings. What is sought after are emotional reactions.

You feed off of what they give you, and you bend them to your will to provide for more food. If fear is flagging, you up the ante to invoke greater fear. If they aren't reacting in a way that is satisfactory, you shift that energy until you are able to feed on the reaction. Until you are satisfied. Whatever that takes.

AFTERCARE

Most players who engage in fantasy role play are aware of the importance of aftercare. Aftercare looks very different depending on the play, the players, and what they need in that moment. Of vital importance is never, ever forgetting that the victim is not the only one who needs aftercare—the perpetrator (e.g., the rapist) needs it as well. In some cases, aftercare for the aggressor might be even more critical. Sound crazy? Not at all. Think about the effort it takes to possess someone you care about, strip them of their humanity and power, use them in ways that might not feel consensual—and then it's over and you're left hanging, needing closure, rapprochement, reassurance that the monster you unleashed isn't indicative of who you really are.

I asked Barak how it was, from the rapist's perspective, to return from the state of consensual nonconsent back to a place of trust:

> The situation might not be clearly consensual until the aftercare phase. In the case of a consensually nonconsensual scene, the action often is explicitly brutal and the aftercare might not be present, or even possible, until the refractory period, when there has been some recovery.
>
> Aftercare must not come too soon after the scene is done. That can impact the arc of the scene, and compromise the emotional journey. Conversely, you can't wait too long: if these emotions are left unresolved, the erosion of trust can take root in that vacuum. And it is vitally important for those taking on the roles of perpetrator and victim. It is critical for the victim in the scene to reassure the abuser that they do still feel that connection and trust, because guilt and shame can damage the emotional stability of the person who has just committed these acts that, without consent, would be terrible abuses.

With this in mind, always remember: negotiate, negotiate, negotiate. It doesn't matter whether you've known your scene partner for decades and you are an old hand in the dungeon. Take the time to foresee and discuss the possibility of negative fallout. Have a Plan B and a Plan C. Play with people you trust, who know and understand what you are up to, and with whom you have discussed your intentions. It can be helpful to line up an "aftercare buddy." An aftercare buddy can be a friend or partner specifically *not* involved in the scene who is prepared to provide interim connection for the participants until they are ready to reconnect and check in. With the help of the buddy, the partners will be able to process whatever might have been unearthed during this journey to the dark side of fantasy.

PLAYING WITH HATE

While there can be an overtly sexual aspect to a rape play scene, there are other dark role plays that may not be explicitly sexual but carry their own unique risks. These are scenes that deal with hate crimes, play that involves the degradation or exploitation of a participant based on their perceived membership in a social group, usually defined by race, religion, sexual orientation, disability, class, ethnicity, nationality, age, gender, gender identity, social status, or political affiliation.

That's a broad, almost limitless palette from which to draw ammunition for some fucked-up scenarios, no? I understand that you may think, Hey, there's nothing out there for me to subject myself to that might fit into a scary, dark scene. I call shenanigans. Are you a wealthy heterosexual white man? Then you might find yourself in a bad way if you fell into the clutches of a female supremacist bent on vengeance, full of disgust and scorn for your worthless, useless excuse for genitals and your grotesque white male privilege. Again, it is all about expanding your definition of what is risky, what is edgy, and personalizing the depersonalization.

In a group discussion about taboo play once, an individual who self-identified as transgendered hesitantly revealed a fantasy they'd had of coordinating a scene that would enact a "fag bashing." This person wanted to experience an eroticized version of being mocked, abused, assaulted, and sexually violated *because of their perceived gender*. This was an especially nuanced exploration for them, they explained, as their affect is often fluid and they embrace a mercurial approach to gender and how they define it. Their hesitation was understandable: they were revealing this highly taboo fantasy in a room full of strangers. While I strive to create a space that is safe for people to share this dark matter, you can never know how other people will react to such revelations. As we expanded the discussion to include this type of play, we talked about risks and how one might approach broaching this topic with a potential play partner. I looked around the room and saw several attendees evincing gleams of recognition and nodding their heads vigorously. I addressed the room: "Hey, anyone else here think this sounds hot, dirty, shocking, fucked up, edgy, *awesome?*" At least a dozen hands shot up, to the surprised delight of the person who had so shyly revealed themselves. "I suggest you start taking numbers, I think you have some planning to do!" I said. We laughed, and dove in further.

I have a friend who uses a wheelchair who shocked the hell out of a roomful of jaded perverts by enacting the victim in a scene where he was kicked out of his chair, dragged around, degraded, and humiliated with all manner of shocking epithets and completely inappropriate language. Yeah, that is pretty fucked up. But the point is, he wanted that experience in order to feel that he is a survivor. From the ashes of such debasement he can rise and feel even stronger and more empowered than before. Once you've had the snot beaten out of you and been called a "crippled faggot gimp" and survived, it can be very empowering to take back the power of those words over you.

Revealing your dark fantasies is risky, yes. But if you do not, you all but zero out your chances of realizing your desires. I struggled for years with memories of a cacophony of conflicts after I discovered my curiosity about pushing the boundaries of sexual consent. As I embarked on a quest to explore my demons, I had to scrape off layer upon layer of guilt and shame before I was clear enough to free my own mind. For me, daring to stare into the face of racism, classism, and sexism and discover why they tripped my erotic triggers was the key to finding a profound level of personal authenticity.

Let's be honest: the majority of us struggle, at some point, with self-esteem. It can be crippling to have our fears reinforced by hate. Suppose you were in a scenario where a partner is belittling you for being Mexican, or queer, Irish Catholic, or Muslim, or short, or fat, a redhead, a Jew, a man, a woman, intersex—for being *different* just because you are you. But what if you realized that these words didn't have the power over you that you thought they did? What if you were able to weather this abuse, this ugliness, and walk away unscathed? Or stronger? What if you were able to look upon your abuser thereafter with compassion instead of rage?

And for those who might take up the mask of the evil villain, think how liberating it would be to revel in those wicked thoughts—thoughts that all of us have entertained. It is not acceptable, in our current social climate, to judge people based on their appearance, to want to take them down, dehumanize them, plunder their body, feed off their fear, consume their energy. But through taboo role play you can. You can let this demon out to play, and acknowledge that these thoughts and feelings do not, in fact, make you a monster. They make you human. You can view yourself with more compassion, knowing that this wickedness is not the totality of your being, even when you indulge your terrifying fantasy.

The first time I negotiated and participated in a scene that explicitly included race-based abuse, my main fear wasn't for my safety. It was for the safety of my partner, who was my friend. I wasn't certain how I would react, whether this would be okay, and mostly, whether I would fly off the handle and try to rip his face off. The scene progressed from casual physical dominance to verbal humiliation, racially tinged verbal abuse, and finally a complete onslaught of overwhelming physical force, invasive sexual aggression, and scathing racial slurs. I panicked for a moment, lost and unsure of why I was here, why I'd permitted this terrible thing to happen. I stared up at him with shock and real fear mingling uneasily in my gut. He eyed me with a lustful disgust that froze my skin. Then he leaned in and asked me,

"Are you wet?"

My mouth dropped in shock. There was no way I—

"Because everyone knows how you nigger cunts love to have the shit kicked out of you. And you know I'll have you begging to take my white cock in your mouth, up your ass—anywhere I want it. Won't you."

I started sobbing, confused and crushed and unable to fight anymore. He shoved me harder against the wall, one hand sliding down over my belly and stopping just short of my pussy. I remembered to resist again but this only evoked a tightening of his hand on my throat.

"Let's just see, shall we? Maybe I'm wrong. Maybe you aren't dripping wet and ready to beg me for it. But I doubt it."

I was *certain* I wasn't physically aroused *at all*. I was enraged, terrified, scared, yes, but it was impossible that—

A sharp inhalation of breath into my lungs was the counterpoint to a contemptuous exhalation of breath from his as his fingers slid effortlessly inside me, twisting with a punishing roughness that blurred my vision as I kicked my feet against him. The look in his eyes was fearsomely cold, and for a moment I was not at all sure where my friend had gone.

"Go on, come like the dirty groveling black bitch you are."

And, gods help me, I did. Shocked, overwhelmed, and completely undone. I orgasmed violently as he stared at me impassively.

In the aftermath of the scene, I was truly shocked at how I had reacted in the midst of what seemed like an impossible situation. Several days later, when I could finally talk to my friend again, I told him about the moment when he seemed *really* into it. He smiled "Well, weren't *you*?"

Indeed.

Is it wiring? Are those of us who crave dark play simply different? Or are we just whistling in the dark as we play with our demons, courageous enough to exploit them for our own pleasure and pain? Ultimately it doesn't matter. What matters is that I have the freedom to make choices—that I have the ability to make a decision to live according to my desires, even if they terrify me.

I encourage you, you with unsettling dreams who find your minds slipping into crevasses when you contemplate devious scenarios: let go of judgment. Get dirty and see who you are on the other side of that darkness. The answer might surprise you.

Endnotes

[1] As in my previous chapter, I deliberately use the plural pronouns *they*, *them*, and *their* to refer to singular persons of any gender, in place of "he or she," "him or her," "his or her." Although this is nonstandard grammatical usage, the traditional forms reflect a gender binary to which I do not subscribe.

CHAPTER 19

THE DARK SIDE

JACK RINELLA

Nearly a year ago, a guy from New York cruised me online, seeking to be imprisoned in my dungeon for the rest of his life. He sought degradation, abuse, humiliation, and (to put it mildly) escape from his current reality. In the ensuing months, he and I maintained a sporadic but ongoing dialogue via email.

His communications by email, chat, and phone intrigued me, and I sought to understand where the guy was coming from and how serious his search was. I found him erratic and ambivalent, and he demonstrated cyclical behavior that told me something was wrong. I finally figured out that he was a drug addict who engaged in episodes of physical abuse every four to six weeks.

His mode of operation was to deny his feelings for about a month, until he could no longer resist them. At that point he would get some recreational drugs to boost his courage, find a man or two to abuse him badly, and then slink home. When the drugs had worn off, he forsook such activity until the cravings slowly reentered his mind and he repeated the cycle.

By the time I had figured this out, my curiosity was at a high point, and I wanted to know more about others like him who wished to be so degraded. To be honest, the controlling and sadistic sides of me were aroused as well. What would it be like, I wondered, to own a subhuman creature like this?

I spent many months researching the profiles of men on various online kink networking sites who sought to serve the darkness. Though they used a wide variety of terms, they all wanted one thing: to become objects of degradation and intense control. Their posts included the words *dark*, *satanic*, *objectification*, *filth*, *permanent*, *mutilation*, *scat*, *worship*, and *incarceration*. These posts are examples of what I mean:

> Sick twisted filthy sewer bottom, ashtray, doormat, gutter rat, barn hand and kennel keeper seeks a perverted sewer top.

> Filthy, perverted, twisted, brutal, sadistic, nasty, top, dom, master needed for sewer pig, gutter rat.

> Looking for noose Master, gloved hands or maybe garrote and KO Master. Also into racial play and religious play.

There was, too, another aspect to my curiosity. In recent years I have been struck by the increasing presence of edge play in our BDSM subculture. Everywhere I turn, I see, hear about, or read about another seminar featuring blood play, highly risky behavior, and taboo-breaking practices of all kinds—public fetish behavior that would have been frowned upon 10 years ago has become almost commonplace.

I wondered what it means that our community is becoming increasingly more inclusive of the darker kinds of play. Where does it lead? Where does it end? I found that I couldn't resist exploring these questions, knowing that there were aspects of myself that sought the same darkness, even as the PC Jack resisted such an admission.

So I posted a new and relatively anonymous bio from an invented (though not really far from reality) persona called the Dark Lord:

> Experienced Lord and Master seeks additional property. I seek to be obeyed and worshipped. My primary fetish is control, which I exercise both sexually and sadistically.
>
> I have an exceptionally high libido and the primary objective of my search is to find men who will be used to satisfy my every sexual desire, without limit or hesitation. I seek to transform you into another toy for my pleasure and sexual gratification.
>
> About you:
> You seek a relationship where you will experi-

ence slavery to the utmost, becoming the subhuman property of your Lord and Master.

You know you were born to suck and get fucked regularly and thoroughly. My semen is your food; my piss your drink.

You desire to be subjugated, degraded, dominated, humiliated, and violated so that you thoroughly realize your authentic low-caste self.

You have the courage to experience this abject state, if only for a weekend.

You want to confirm [or deny] through actual experience your inner conviction that you were born for life in this abject state and nothing else will satisfy you until you are completely controlled by your Lord and Master.

You will obey and surrender. Resistance on your part will be met by punishment.

I approach this process as one of testing your suitability to serve me. Show yourself serious and worthy of my attention or go chat with some other poser. Serious applicants may begin the interview process with a message to the Dark Lord that includes an email address, a chat ID, and a phone number. COMPLETE DISCRETION IS ASSURED.

This enslavement may include: Anal penetration and violation, Ashtray slavery, Ass fucking, Begging & pleading, Behavior modification, Bacchanalian celebration, Blasphemy, Bloodletting, Branding, Breath control, Chastity, Chores, Clamps, Cock and ball torture, Cock sucking, Confinement, Crucifixion, Cum control, Cutting, Degradation, Dehumanization, Demasculinization, Deprivation, Dionysian initiation, Domestic service, Encasement, Enforced exercise, Face fucking, Filth, Flogging, Groveling, Hobbling, Humbling, Humiliation, Idolatry, Inferiority, Isolation, Light deprivation, Long-term bondage, Marking, Milking, Nakedness, Obedience, Objectification, Oral invasion, Orgies, Ownership, Pain, Phallic worship, Piercing, Pimping, Piss, Praise and adoration, Predicament bondage, Prescribed dieting, Public display, Punching, Punishment, Raunch, Restraints, Rimming, Scheduling, Sex magic, Service, Shit, Silence, Slapping, Slavery to the Dark Lord, Smoke, Snot, Spit, Subjugation, Submission, Surrender, Suspension, Sweat, Tantric training, Total Control, Violation, Whipping, and Worship of the Dark Lord.

Over six months, I received numerous hits on my profile and a large number of "cruises," where members signaled interest in serving me. To those who did so, I wrote back asking if they were interested in "serving my dark desires." Many replied yes and were invited to apply.

Applying became the standard for evaluating their interest. I asked for their email address, chat ID, and phone number so I could contact them off-site. About 120 men responded with contact information, and it is on my communications with these men that I base the following reflections. (If you were one of these men, let me assure you that my interest was, and still is, genuine. It was more than just a research project.)

GLOSSARY OF TERMS

Over the ensuing months, I found myself in the position of explaining what I, the Dark Lord, meant by several of the terms in my profile. Among them were words we often use but that have troubling implications in our Judaic-Christian society. Let me begin by trying to shed some light on what I mean by some of these terms.

The Dark Side

> Dark: Lacking or having very little light; gloomy; dismal; sullen or threatening; difficult to understand; obscure; concealed or secret; mysterious; lacking enlightenment or culture; exhibiting or stemming from evil characteristics; sinister; absence of light.[1]

For numerous social, religious, and historical reasons the polarity of Light and Dark is often equated with the polarity of Good and Evil. Therefore the "Dark Lord" is immediately identified with Satan, as is the Dark Side.

In nature, both light and dark are neutral phenomena. Only when we enter the realm of morality and theology does the imputation of evil to darkness begin to cause serious problems. If indeed God is everywhere, then God is in the darkness as well as the light. Is Satan really the opposite of God?

Is Satan "outside" of God? I doubt it.

In much of the correspondence the Dark Lord received, there were inquiries into satanic worship. My response was to refer the applicant to Elaine Pagels's excellent book *The Origin of Satan*. This renowned Gnostic scholar shows that Satan is the creation of Hebrew/Christian intolerance of others. I came to the conclusion that I was not a satanist insofar as I refused to worship a creature that I did not believe existed as the caricature depicted in my childhood.

Similarly, I was asked about blasphemy and eternal damnation. It became obvious that most applicants had a strong belief in basic Judaic-Christian paradigms, especially the ones that condemned them to Hell. Over and over again, I saw that both the fantasy and the discussion were in fact based in religion, and unfortunately based on unclear—and unconscious—beliefs.

I also noticed that many terms (some of which I used in my profile above) were relative, interpreted according to the applicants' religious perspective. What is blasphemy, for instance, to one devotee is holiness to another. Muslims think that Hindus are blasphemous idolaters. I don't get the idea that Hindus agree with them.

Worship

Intrinsic in the consideration of darkness is one's spiritual beliefs and understanding of good and evil. Though we don't often state it, an altered state is often akin to a Gnostic revelation. Gnosis is, after all, a theological belief that deity is present in and operates in the human selfhood. The Dark

Lord made it clear in his list of stipulations that he wanted to be worshipped, to literally become the slave's god.

Obedience, then, was seen as obedience to god. The Dark Lord's authority, for the slave, would become pervasive, even complete. The gulf between the exalted Lord and the degraded slave would become—what? Infinite? Where does this god trip lead? What does the extreme nature of this polarity create in terms of the power exchange?

These questions might seem preposterous, but they are not out of order to those who are seriously involved in master/slave relationships. On occasion, a slave has admitted to worshipping his or her master or a master has admitted to having a godlike relationship with his or her slave.

It is easy to dismiss such practices by saying, "Oh, they don't really mean God with a capital G." But it is clear that for some, "the Lord" is not Jehovah, Jesus, or Allah, or any of the other gods of traditional worship.

The Unconscious

When we look at the polarity of light and dark in terms of the known and the unknown, we find ourselves in the realm of what is conscious and what is unconscious. It is not an unfamiliar analogy; we are all cognizant of the phrase "the heart of darkness," popularized by a novel of that title by Joseph Conrad. What evil, after all, lurks in the heart of man?

> *It is obvious that even as players flout some taboos, other taboos remain that are too kinky for most of us and that, therefore, we will not violate.*

My reading of Jungian psychology has given me some ideas about what it is that we do in the BDSM community. As I see it, the intent of BDSM is to transport both the bottom and the top to an altered state of consciousness, though it certainly can mean other things to other players. There are many terms for the mind trip: an out-of-body experience, "going deep," for the bottom, *subspace*, for the top, *top space*. Whatever name you give it, it is an often-sought but rarely achieved trip of extraordinary bliss, joy, and peace. In scholarly literature it has been referred to as an altered state of consciousness (ASC).

Though most players are satisfied with (dare I say it?) "conventional" fetishes such as flogging, whipping, and fisting as a way to enter an altered state, the Dark Lord's applicants expressed a desire to progress to more intensive activities, such as blood play, extreme pain, degradation, and scat.

It is obvious that even as players flout some taboos, other taboos remain that are too kinky for most of us and that, therefore, we will not violate. The Dark Lord's exploration raises the question "Where do we draw the line?"

Yet are there really any lines to cross in the mind? What darkness lurks in the depth of one's unconscious self? How do we integrate that darkness in our lives to become whole persons? Or do we do so at all?

Limits

The most difficult part of my exploration of the Dark Lord was the question of limits. In light of the extreme nature of some of these desires, what were my own limits? How far was I willing to go? Would I, for instance, allow a partner

> *I believe that one of the most important benefits of BDSM is that it creates a space and a community where we can safely explore the deep longings of our soul, where we can be the sissy maid or slave or pirate or top or lady we long to be.*

to worship Satan, eat my shit, or languish in darkness while chained to a cold stone wall in my dungeon?

How do you answer these questions when faced with an email such as this: "SIR, it knows it was predisposed for a life of slavery under your control. It knows it is ready to surrender its worthless pathetic self in submission and obedience to your will, helping it to obtain deeper actualization of its true slave nature as it satisfies your every command. Its innermost need is to submit 100% of its mind, body, soul, and spirit/ego. It is ready!"

I believe that one of the most important benefits of BDSM is that it creates a space and a community where we can safely explore the deep longings of our soul, where we can be the sissy maid or slave or pirate or top or lady we long to be. Is it so unlikely that the same subculture could allow us to be the shit-slave toilet, the degraded object, or the worthless subhuman?

As we say, "It's only kinky when you don't do it." How can we label something as "too extreme" when what we do every day is labeled just that way by mainstream society?

In the end I did come up with limits: I wouldn't do anything that was illegal. I would not spread disease or inflict physical harm that would necessitate a doctor's care. I would not allow an applicant to become financially dependent upon me.

Those limits were generally acceptable to most applicants,

though several of them refused to continue the conversation when they figured out that the Dark Lord would require them to pay room and board and to have health insurance. "I'm the Dark Lord," I wrote more than once, "not a jail keeper or a sugar daddy."

Others ended the dialogue when I refused to entertain their need for intoxicants to undergo their fantasy. I am a firm believer in experiencing fetish to the fullest, rather than using drugs or alcohol to mitigate its effects. I have also found that drug-using slaves are useless when it come to service of any kind, and the Dark Lord demands to be served. It is all about the Dark Lord's desires—they must come first.

Desire

> Desire: To wish or long for; want. To express a wish for; request. A wish or longing. A request or petition. The object of longing. Sexual appetite; passion.[2]

I have long held the belief that not every fantasy is meant to become a reality. We must decide which fantasies can be lived and which cannot. The track records of those 120 applicants made my decision-making process a lot easier than one would expect.

Of the 120 applicants, some 15 are still showing interest, and about half of those are of more recent acquaintance. As with most cruising, the majority have simply failed to respond to the emails, chats, or phone calls I initiated in an effort to continue a dialogue. Few ever got to the point of seeing my dungeon. Some, to their credit, ended the conversation politely, giving such reasons as "You're too old for me," "I have to beg off due to family problems," and "I'm not really into the raunch and worship you seek." These results are the same I've found with cruising in general.

But I think there is an unspoken message in this as well. When faced with the possible reality of our deepest desires, their desirability fades quickly. We allow other choices to take precedence over the darkest of our dreams.

There seems to be a contradiction here that probably derives from poorly defined terminology. How, for instance, can an "object" object to the age of its owner? Could a chair or a goldfish do this? I think not. It is only when the full effect and the extent of the objectification dawns on us that we see what appears to be its intrinsic impossibility. Would any of these cybercruisers, after all, be willing to actually live in a dungeon without access to the Internet?

Control

In my 28 years as a practicing leatherman I have learned much about myself and my desires. I've come to the conclusion that my primary fetish is control, which is certainly exercised through other fetishes, especially those involving pain and bondage. As my profile made clear, the overriding characteristic I sought from an applicant was obedience. I wanted to be in control.

The conundrum I repeatedly encountered was that applicants would make requirements that allowed them to maintain some kind of control. So I had men who wanted everything I offered but who, for example, refused to provide for their own upkeep.

It seems to me that the control issue fundamentally stems from instinctual reactions (see Maslow's hierarchy of needs) that we have little likelihood of overcoming, self-preservation being the most obvious of them. Ceding complete control to another is much too dangerous for the psyche to allow, unless the control is limited by factors that render it less than complete.

The only plausible path out of this contradiction is to create a deep bond of trust between the "object" and his or her Lord. I wonder, though, if this bond, as necessary as it is, might not then pose another difficulty: that this trust mitigates or eradicates the polarity in such a way that domination and subjugation, in their most intense forms, lose their power and effect.

Repression and Expression

The great value of our BDSM subculture, I believe, is that it creates the conditions for us to experiment with desire without limit, judgment, or exception. The key word here is *experiment*. Experimentation often means just dabbling—that is, entertaining a thought without necessarily executing it fully. Our community is in the fortunate position of being able to express to an extent and therefore experience to an extent aspects of ourselves of which we are only partly conscious. This allows us the opportunity to experience the deepest darkness, neither repressing nor expressing it, while being able to assess its meaning and implications.

Even given what little experience I was able to gain of the more extreme activities in the Dark Lord's profile, I found considerable information about the meaning of darkness, of perversion, and of authenticity. That information can best be summed up as realizing that we can see the dark side, admit to it, learn something about it and about ourselves, without necessarily embracing or becoming what we might desire.

Yes, I saw self-destruction in the motivation of some who sought refuge, degradation, or punishment in the Dark Lord's dungeon. I have seen "Dark Lords" act irresponsibly as well. More often, though, I found men who were seeking to unravel the complexity of their desires while intuitively, if not explicitly, holding on to the more fundamental necessity of self-preservation and healthy activity.

ABOUT THE DARK LORD

In the final analysis, this exploration was more about myself than about my applicants. Though the conversation continues with a few men who are seeking a more intense form of slavery, the fruitlessness of the search leads me to question its validity and viability. I have also had to evaluate how real my desire was to become the Dark Lord.

Patrick, my slave and partner of more than 15 years, commented recently that my failure to attract a viable "object" rested within myself. It was just not part of my nature, he thought, to engage in the kind of dehumanization, humiliation, and degradation that being the Dark Lord required. My discussions with applicants led them to see that I lacked the ego, the necessary haughtiness, to pull off the role successfully. I was just too friendly, too kind, to be that dark.

A recent scene with one of the applicants I continue to have contact with illustrates my personal conundrum. The man in question vacillates between wanting degradation and avoiding it. When, after four months of nearly talking the idea to death, he arrived to try a week in my dungeon, he was well guarded by a list of limits I had agreed to, many of which left control in his hands, not mine. The fundamental issue was his inability to trust me. I couldn't tie him to an immovable object, for instance—chain him to the wall in the dungeon or to a cross. It was obvious that putting him in a cage for the night was out of the question until he knew me better.

Could I have simply violated his limits and tied him up anyway? I think I could have. Would the Dark Lord have done so? Certainly. Would I have? Not then and there, and probably never. Should I have? Ah, there's the question, since I certainly wanted to. Darkness, it would seem, lurks in my heart just as fully as in any other.

NEXT

Having enjoyed and learned from the Dark Lord experience, I will continue it, adapting my approach to the lessons I learned. There'll be less compromise and more authority in my words and actions. As for its fruitfulness, or lack thereof, I will most likely spend less attention on it, except for those candidates who indeed show some process of developing a relationship with me.

I have come to the conclusion that if I am to realize my Dark Lord fantasy, I have to act as the Dark Lord would. I cannot be "Jack" and "Dark" at the same time. Only time will tell if I can become the Dark Lord. On the other hand, time has made it obvious that I want to do so. I want to see where this ends. If and when it does, I'm sure there'll be another story to tell.

Endnotes

1   Definition of dark, www.thefreedictionary.com/dark.
2   Definition of desire, www.thefreedictionary.com/desire.

CHAPTER 20

MINDFUCK (C'MON, DOES IT NEED ANY OTHER TITLE?)
EDGE

My name is Edge, and I mindfuck. Oh, I do *lots* of other things—beat the crap out of faggots,[1] feed smoke to stogiepigs, throw some mean Japanese rope bondage, hell, I even cuddle (though only with my cub)—but mindfuck is what I'm most known for because, really, it's what I do best. Dunno how, dunno why. Just a knack, ya know? I mean, give me a singletail and I'm a total klutz; I'll have it wrapped around my neck somehow in minutes. Give me a TENS unit and I'll end up crossing some wires and shorting the whole thing out. Give me a set of needles and I'll gently place them back down. But give me one hour—just *one* hour—with you, alone in a room, and you *will* know what mindfuck is. And you will *not* forget. Not a promise, not a threat, just a fact. But, shit, you're there and I'm here so this essay is gonna have to do.

Read on. Get wet. Get hard. Get scared. Get excited. Get it. It's *good*.

Before we get into the meat of the matter, though, I have a few warnings. First, this isn't an essay that teaches technique. There is no cookie-cutter mindfuck, really—no single thing you can do with everyone. That's what makes mindfuck so powerful and really so intimate. My goal here is to introduce you to some of the dynamics in this kind of scene, to give you some sense of the process. Second, because you're often playing with fear, which risks panic, this can be a kind of edge play. Third, I'm revealing secrets of the trade in this essay, so stop reading if that spoils it for you. It's a bit like knowing the secrets behind a magician's tricks. Knowing how the illusion works either 1) spoils it for you, 2) makes it that much easier for you to volunteer to be sawed in half, or 3) helps you enjoy the magic that much more because you can appreciate the skill of the sleight of hand. If it's going to spoil it for you, stop reading and go get mindfucked. Finally, I'm going to sound like a psycho killer at times. I am not. Promise.

WHAT THE FUCK?

Assuming you're still reading, let's start by thinking about just what mindfuck is and isn't. There are any number of ways we might define mindfuck: playing with someone's head, edge play with consciousness, consensual hallucination (which is why mindfuck works so nicely in cyberspace), erotic terrorism, sexual lying, or perhaps even a theater of intimacy.

But there's one definition I tend to use the most because I think it best describes what happens in a mindfuck scene: *Mindfuck is making someone think something is happening that isn't really happening.*

What do I mean by that? Well, mindfuck can cover a broad spectrum of activities, ranging from the rather mild to the extremely wild. For example, a rather mild mindfuck would be tying up and blindfolding your partner and then making her think you've left or that someone else has arrived. An edgier example would be starting a scene by making someone write his suicide note at gunpoint. (And, yes, I've done that one. Always tear up the first note and tell them it's not convincing enough. Be sure to obtain samples of their signature well before the scene so that you can confirm they're not faking that part either. Doesn't hurt to make them dig their own grave, too. Just saying.)

There are many things mindfuck isn't, even though it often gets bound up, mixed up, and confused with those other things. For example, mindfuck isn't always edge play. Edge play is pushing the envelope of a scene—any scene. So edge play for you may include very risky activities, like breath control and weapon sex, but really, every scene has its own edge: plaster bondage is an edge form of bondage, double fisting is an edge form of fisting, singletail whipping is an edge form of flailing. So, while a lot of mindfucks *can* be edge play, they don't have to be. Conversely, most edge play doesn't involve mindfuck at all.

Mindfuck isn't playing head games, though you might think of head games as a kind of nonconsensual mindfuck.

"Game players" (and they're all over cyberspace) are creating that sense of illusion and are, essentially, lying, but not in a way that works for both players. Clearly, the person doing the lying is getting something out of it, maybe getting off on it, but the person being lied to has not *agreed* to be lied to. That's not to say that head game players are not into mindfuck, but it is a way to further delineate what makes mindfuck mindfuck. One of its essential elements is the mysterious and intoxicating paradox of consensual nonconsent. Consensual nonconsent can be summarized like this: *I'm going to lie to you all throughout the mindfuck but only 'cause you've told me it's okay to fuck with your head like that*. To put it simply, mindfuck always requires the consent of all parties involved.

> *Mindfuck isn't mind control. Mindfuck is making someone believe something is happening that isn't really happening.*

Mindfuck isn't mind control. Mindfuck is making someone believe something is happening that isn't really happening; mind control is making someone believe something is happening that really *is* happening. With mindfuck, trust is used to enter and then leave this altered sense of what is real. With mind control, trust is used to enter and then make permanent this altered sense of what is real. The two work very well together and are often combined, but they're definitely not the same thing.

Finally, mindfuck isn't interrogation. I often see mindfuck and interrogation paired in classes at various SM educational events, but there's a crucial difference—you *know* the interrogation isn't real: you're not really a prisoner of war and your Top doesn't really work for the Gestapo, you're not really a perp and your Top isn't really a cop (well, unless you're really, really lucky). It's the sense of could-be-real-but-hope-it-isn't that defines mindfuck for me, and that's something that doesn't happen in interrogation scenes. Besides, you know how to end an interrogation scene: give up the right info. For a bottom in a mindfuck scene, half the fun is not knowing how, when, or *whether* it will end.

Given what mindfuck is and isn't, any scene can use mindfuck but some scenes seem particularly good for it. In particular, scenes that might seem difficult to do "for real" make sense for mindfuck, since mindfuck can make extreme situations feel real. I'm talking about scenes like kidnapping, white slavery, rape, castration, even snuff. Whoa—extreme examples, I know, but if you're the kind of person who has desires like these, mindfuck comes in very handy.

WHY THE FUCK?

So why the fuck do people get into mindfuck? For one thing, there's a good biological reason. In the kink scene there are a lot of endorphin junkies, often called pain pigs. They get a real, actual physical high from pain because the brain releases its own natural painkillers. In the same way, mindfuckers can be considered adrenaline junkies. Fear triggers the fight-or-flight response, fueled by adrenaline, which, as it turns out, is chemically related to amphetamines. Granted, it's a very different kind of high for mindfuckers: not a mellow, floaty "my vulva is one with the universe" high but a jittery, revved-up "oh fuck oh fuck oh fuck" kind of high. Endorphins are like great downers but adrenaline is uppers all the way. And it's just as addictive. Don't believe me? Go ask anyone who likes to jump off bridges or out of airplanes.

For others, though, part of the appeal of mindfuck is its potential for magic. One way to define magic is to say that it is the ability to alter someone's perception of reality. In that sense, mindfuck literally is a kind of magic because during the mindfuck things feel very real. Thus it can be used for very transformative, spiritual, cathartic, shamanic scenes: walking someone through death or trauma, for example. I've used mindfuck a lot for catharsis. I helped one boy through the loss of his Daddy on 9/11 and a woman deal with the fact that her family had deliberately forgotten her grandfather because he didn't get out of Germany in time during the Holocaust. Powerful, magical shit it is.

But for the more jaded among us (me included) mindfuck is about a special kind of fear—the fear and wonder we had when we first got into kink. Let's face it, at first kink is mysterious and unreadable and even a little scary, but it becomes prosaic, if not boring. You know what they say: it's only kinky the first time. My cock used to drip just seeing a pair of cheap handcuffs, but these days I need the most elaborate restraints devised by the most devious minds just to get my attention. That kinda sucks. Mindfuck brings back the edge—the edge is where we teetered before exploring kink, before we stepped into this world. I can remember my first few scenes. My heart would be racing, my stomach flip-flopping. Nerves, fear, adrenaline. It's nice to feel that way again once you've gotten inured to it all.

And as with most forms of SM, people get off on mindfuck because it plays so well with power. The bottom experiences an enormous sense of being controlled, because someone is "in your head." Mindfuck goes beyond physical control and reaches into the psyche, where it feels much more real. And *fuckkkkk*, what a rush for the Top to feel that kind of power and control.

Add it all up, and you can see that mindfuck also lets us experience outlaw SM. Safe, sane, consensual, risk-aware consensual kink—blah blah blah. Mindfuck lets you do all the stuff you're not supposed to do. You're not *supposed* to rape people. You're not *supposed* to kill them. You're not *supposed* to offer their souls to Satan in return for more power and pleasure. You're only *supposed* to play nice—hard maybe, but still nice. Mindfuck lets you play nasty, though again only through consensual nonconsent.

THE 3 F'N MFS

I know a lot of my examples tend to the edgy side of mindfuck (look at my name, for Christ's sake) but there are whole other categories of mindfuck to consider. And thanks to my enormous anal-retentiveness, I've categorized three types of mindfucks. I call these the "3 F'n MFs."

Fear-Based

Fear-based mindfucks involve scenes that derive their erotic energy from fear. And yeah, these are the kinds of mindfucks I do, primarily. For example, playing with weapons is a fear-based mindfuck. The gun could be real—but it doesn't have to be to get the same charge. The fear's the thing, and fear is inherent to the scene. It drives the play and it gets the players off.

Fantasy-Based

Fantasy-based mindfucks involve scenes that may not contain elements of fear but rather transmutations that cannot happen in reality. For example, there are folks out there with microphilia and macrophilia—fantasies of shrinking to the size of a toy or growing into a giant. That's not something you can do for real, but it is something you can approximate with mindfuck. I've also run across more than one man who fantasizes about being turned into a cigar. Again, can't actually make it happen, but since mindfuck makes you think something's happening that isn't, it can help a pig explore these kinds of unrealizable desires.

Faith-Based

Now, technically faith-based mindfucks should be called "trust-based," but then it wouldn't be the "3 F'n MFs" and I'm not only anal-retentive but also hungry for symmetry. These are mindfucks that eroticize not fear or fantasy but trust. They involve tests of service, submission, and trust and can be used to deepen the relationship between a Master or Mistress and a slave. Imagine a scene that starts with a Mistress asking

"How far are you willing to go for me?" and you can imagine where mindfuck can take two people. My favorite example isn't sexual but it is from the Bible. (Blasphemous, I know, but that kinda turns me on.) God tells Abraham, "Hey, go kill yer son Isaac for me" and Abraham just about does it, then God says, "Nah, I was just mindfucking you." Classic!

There's also one category of antimindfuck. This is something you should not play with ever, period. *Do not ever mindfuck around someone's phobias.* Why? Phobias are by definition irrational fears; irrational fears provoke panic; and panic is dangerous for everyone in the scene. I have a great story to illustrate what I mean. I played with a boy once who told me about a scene he had with some other Top. The guy had the boy in leather restraints chained to a bed. He also knew the boy had arachnophobia, fear of spiders. So Mr. Dumbass Top decides to take out his pet tarantula and put it on the restrained boy's chest. The boy reported to me that tarantulas make a popping sound when they hit the wall. (He broke through the restraints.)

Drowning's the one for me. You can do a lot of shit to me, but since I almost drowned when I was a kid you play around with that *at all* and I'm gonna freak and then take it out on you. So, no phobias—agreed?

FUCKIN' RULES

It should be pretty clear by now that mindfuck is a huge fucking category with lots of room for all kinds of kinksters to do all kinds of things. But there are some basic rules to keep in mind to help any kind of mindfuck happen.

Rule One: Control the Info

The Top, by definition, has to know more about the scene than the bottom. This starts with a balance of communication and mystery. The bottom has to know what's going to happen but also know that he doesn't know everything that's going to happen, or how it's going to happen. The bottom has to know the Top enough to trust her, but not so much that she feels *fully* safe. There needs to be some lingering doubt, always, and always carefully managed. I like to say that *the bottom should only trust you enough to show up for the scene.*

So as the Mindfucker you have to know if the gun is loaded, and the bottom can't know. (You have to know if the gun is real, too, and the bottom can't know.) You have to know if you're going to kill that person, and the bottom can't know. You have to know how it will end, and the bottom can't know.

This also means that you have to know what your bottom knows. I've done a bit of weaponsex and I always get hard shoving the barrel of my 9 mm Beretta 92FS down some hungry pig's throat. But I ain't an idiot. The gun I use is 1) a realistic blank-firing replica and 2) never loaded. But a smart pig who's done a lot of gunsex is gonna suck on that barrel when it's in his mouth. Why? Get plenty of air, there's no bullet in the chamber, so you know it's not loaded (or at least not chambered). All the fear goes away and, heck, that ain't much fun. So, if I know I'm playing with a pig who knows how to do that, man, I just plug up that barrel with a bit of cotton. I can see the fear in their eyes when their clever little trick sends them a whole different message, the message I want them to have in their heads.

That's because "Control the Info" means more than *just* "controlling" information; it means managing the information a bottom has access too. Innuendo, sensory control, half-truths—they all play a part. In this sense, a blindfold is your best friend, because the brain is used to processing visual information. Slap a blindfold on anyone, and I mean *anyone*, and the mindfuck has started. Their brain just runs with the last visual input it got and then tries to extend it. So, you see me with a big fucking hunting knife and then I blindfold you. Your brain still sees that knife and not the little wooden toothpick I'm poking at your privates. Information managed. Same thing with sound, once someone's blindfolded. Get 'em tied, get 'em sightless, walk away, slam the door. They're going to think you left. They won't know, of course, but it's that not knowing that makes the mindfuck happen.

Rule Two: Less Is More
The mindfuck isn't happening out here in the real world, though it might look that way. Instead, the mindfuck is always happening up in the bottom's head. So the Mindfucker needs to get the bottom to do the bulk of the work up in there. That means you don't want to overdo anything in the scene; instead, you need to provide the context for the bottom to activate the scene. For example, one very bad mindfuck scene I was in was a kidnapping back in my bottoming days that was just, well, melodramatic. After the guy "kidnapped"

me (by which I mean I had to help him drag me over to the waiting van), he "called" someone and said something along the lines of "I've got him. Erase all his information." Oy. I knew it was only going to go downhill from there because it was suddenly very obvious just how not real this kidnapping was. The Top did too much, went too far.

Best way to follow the Less Is More rule? *Confirm nothing.* I once totally mindfucked this bootlicker online. He was convinced, and I mean utterly convinced, that I was controlling his mind. The chats went something like this:

"Oh, fuck, Sir, you're in my head, aren't you?"

"Am I?"

"Shit, I knew it. Fuck, what are you doing to me?"

"Wouldn't you like to know." I didn't have to do anything. I didn't even really have to lie to him about what was going on. I just had to hold back and let his head fuck itself. Sweet.

Rule Three: Deliver and Maintain

As a Top you need to deliver the mindfuck and maintain it; otherwise the spell will be broken. That means reading where the bottom is, doing what it takes to maintain the illusion, but also knowing when it's coming to a head and timing the scene appropriately. Every lie has its limits. You need to know those limits and tweak the dynamic to keep the sense of unreality real. For example, you get all jazzed and jizzed thinking about me drugging and raping you, so when you show up I shove a pill down your throat (maybe make you wash it down with my piss). Now, at first, you're gonna think it's all happening. And, soon, you're going to feel a little weird and probably a little tired. I mean, fuck, we're *all* tired these days, so no wonder, right? But sooner or later you're going to realize you're not passing out. That lie has a definite limit.

THE FUCKING SAFETY VALVE

All these rules support one goal: for the Top to get the bottom to the point where she can say up in her head, *I know I'm safe and this isn't real, but what if it is?* I call this the safety valve because it allows the bottom to control the amount of fear he wants to experience. Not excited enough? Let yer head drift over to the *What if it is real?* side. Starting to freak out? Slide back down to *I'm safe and this isn't real*.

This safety valve mechanism is crucial for a successful mindfuck. If you leave out either part of it, it all falls to shit. If the bottom is sitting there only thinking the first part, *I'm safe and this isn't real*, then there's no fear, no fulfillment of fantasy, no test of faith. It's just another scene. Fun, maybe, hot, maybe, but just another scene where we're all safe and playing hard but nice. At the same time, fuck, you're screwed if all you remember is the second part, *but what if it is?* If the bottom gets stuck on the idea that it's all real, you risk real panic. And panic, let me say again, is a really, really bad thing in a scene.

The good news is that it's not that hard to get the valve working. That's what the rules are for. Control the Info to leave enough doubt to activate both sides. Remember that Less Is More, and the bottom's head can do all the work, sliding up and down the scale of fear as needed. Deliver and

Maintain, and everyone involved can ride that mindfuck for as long as you all want.

SOME FUCKING METHODS

Part of what the rules remind us is that all mindfuck is really self-mindfuck. If you've done any play with hypnosis, this might be familiar to you. All hypnosis is self-hypnosis, all mind control is self–mind control. As a mindfucking Top, all you need to do and all you want to do is create the context for this self-persuasion to happen. I've got a few methods to help you out with that.

First: Ask questions that prompt contextualized thinking. Ask questions that get the bottom's head in the right place. For example, in a fear-based mindfuck you might have a verbal script peppered with questions like "Who will miss you most when you die? Will they remember you? Did you say goodbye? Did you say you're sorry?" In a fantasy-based mindfuck you might be asking, "How will it feel to be turned into a cigar? Do you ever think about what it would feel like to be lit? To feel the heat consuming you?" And in a faith-based mindfuck, the questions are serious shit: "Will you trust me with your life? Will you do anything for me?" Ask the question, and the bottom's brain takes over. It answers it. It fills in the gaps. It makes the magic happen.

I call my second recommended method "LILO," which stands for "lie in; lie out." (Any coders out there reading this? Recognize it? Remember GIGO?) This one's pretty simple: if you manipulate the information going into the brain, it will make decisions consistent with that information. Obviously this method has a lot to do with both the Control the Info and Less Is More rules. Manipulating sight and sound is part of this technique, but it also involves useful lies like using a replica gun, switching their clothes for larger clothes in a shrinking scene, or just holding something sharp on the balls. Here's my favorite example of LILO. I did this mindfuck class once where I pulled a victim from the audience and had her holding a small baggie with a little stick in it. I told the whole class about my recent experience with poison ivy (true), read aloud a whole bunch of shit about how nasty and pervasive the active ingredient is (true), talked about how it fucking drove me crazed to feel that itching (true). Then I put on rubber gloves and took out the stick, holding it very, very close to my victim's skin. She was freaking out, especially when I finally touched her tits with it. Only then did I tell her it was some twig I had found outside the hotel—not poison ivy at all. Lie in; lie out.

Finally (and easiest of all), use silence. Silence just about equals mindfuck. It can be eerie, discomforting, and disturbing. For one thing, it deprives the brain of aural information. For another, we all know someone's guilty when they plead the Fifth. Remember, the *real* psycho killer doesn't tell it to rub the lotion on its skin. The real one doesn't say anything at all. Just looks at you. Freaky fearful fun, that.

THE FUCKING DYNAMIC

Now, the easiest way to put together all these rules and

methods is to think of mindfuck as a kind of theater or performance sex. This means you need to think about plot, setting, props, characters, movement, and climax.

Plot's a biggie because every mindfuck has a plot. The plot guides the events, structures the dynamic, and suggests the arc of the scene. The plot needs to be discussed but not scripted—there should always be room for improvisation. What's great about plot is that we live in a culture of stories. That means that for any given plot in any given mindfuck the bottom already knows how it ends. And, because they do, that's where their head goes. The moment you invade their home, they're thinking about the rape. The moment you pull out the gun, they've already been shot. Thus any plot can be used to "make them mindfuck themselves." But more basically, the plot lays out the scene.

Setting is important, too, but dammit, setting is tricky, because it's often hard to get it *authentic*. For example, I don't know how things are where you live, but by me all the best abandoned warehouses have already been converted into very trendy lofts. When it comes to setting, sometimes you just have to do the best you can—and sometimes that turns out to be even better. For example, I once played with this Jewish guy who wanted to be the kike to my Nazi. I thought about investing in the big swastika flag and all that; I even looked at a few online. But man, I knew if I bought that online my name would end up on some interesting lists—not just with the government but with some scary-assed companies. So, instead, I printed out a bunch of pages from White Power websites and highlighted some key passages. When the kike arrived, this material was lying on the coffee table. And you know what? It worked even better. Let's face it, Nazis today don't live in some freaking Reichstag. They live in apartments and condos and suburban houses. It ended up being a more realistic setting and the scene was fucking *hot*. Less Is More, you see?

Depending on the mindfuck, props can be really important too. Sometimes these are easy. Want someone to think you're making them shrink? Give them clothes to wear at the start of the scene and have the exact outfit two sizes larger waiting for them at the end of the scene (all tags ripped out, of course). In a case like that, props make the scene. In all cases, consider what would be appropriate, and then also consider what can be approximated. Like good theater, believing can make something real. For example, one year at IML this guy in the lobby was totally freaking because a bud of mine was in uniform and had a plastic gun. The guy knew it was plastic but it still freaked him out. Control the Info, my friends. Replica guns look and feel very real. (They're great for pistol-whipping, too.)

I'm a sick bastard so one of my favorite props is a body bag. I don't mean a bondage bag or a sleepsack. I mean a *body bag*—you know, the kind they put your corpse in so that your decaying juices won't get all over the place. What do I do with it? Nothing, really. I just leave it out. Let them see it. If they ask about it, I change the subject. Control the Info. Less Is More. (Told you I'd sound like a psycho killer. I'm not, really.)

If you're the Top you're also going to need to develop a character. This is like role play, with one minor, *crucial* difference: the Top is playing a role but the bottom absolutely cannot be. They just have to be themselves, because if they feel as if they're playing a role they know it's not real. But the Mindfucker needs to be *absolutely* convincing, and sometimes that means thinking inside the bottom's head and then beyond it. Let me tell you about the psycho killer. He's not angry; he doesn't yell. That's not how to freak out a bottom. Instead, the psycho killer is perfectly calm—a little *too* calm, if you know what I mean. Fucks them up every time.

I should point out that characters play a role primarily in fear-based mindfucks. In some fantasy-based ones, both of you might be playing a character. In faith-based ones, neither of you should, since it's all about bringing trust and submission to a whole new level.

True for all mindfucks, though, is that you need movement (or development) and a climax: the scene has to be going somewhere. It might be someplace the bottom knows, or not. For example, in a castration scene, you're clearly building up to a climax. How fast do you want to move to it? Whatcha gonna do when you get there? As the Top, you should plan these elements in advance and then direct the scene like a theater director.

FUCKING: BEFORE, DURING, AFTER
Before
Before any mindfuck you need to have communication. As a Top, you need to know what the bottom's trip is and what makes their trip their trip. As a bottom, you need to think about the details. So you want to be kidnapped. Okay, but

how? Grabbed and put in a van? Chloroformed? Spiked drink? The details make *all* the difference. The information should flow mostly one way, of course (see Rule One) but this communication is vital for the bottom too. Does this Top "get" you and your scene? Does she get your head space? You have to know before you show up.

And showing up takes some trust. Fuck, any good scene takes trust. In a mindfuck there needs to be some core of trust—but *just* enough. As I said before, there should be just enough trust for both parties to show up and start things off. More than that and it's just going to get in the way. Now, sufficient communication will go a long way in building this trust, but different bottoms will need different levels of assurance. Of course the exception here is the faith-based mindfuck, which is all about trust, which builds on trust already in place.

The last thing you need to do before a mindfuck is have a plan. Spontaneous mindfucks are possible (just run into me at the bar and find out), but the better ones, the more elaborate ones, take some time, some thought, and often a lot of planning. The Top may need to gather specific resources; if nothing else, she should be planting suggestions about what may or may not happen in the bottom's mind.

During
During the scene different parties have different things to do. Tops: Assume your character and stay in it. Be schizoid, too. That is, one part of your brain has to be all in psycho killer mode (or for a fantasy-based mindfuck, mad scientist mode);

the other part of your brain needs to be sane, needs to monitor both the bottom *and* that other psycho part of the brain in play. Remember, you can't stop and check in with a bottom in a mindfuck: "Are you okay? Am I raping you hard enough? Is this gun too scary? Should I put it away?" Ugh. Scene ruined. Being schizoid is the only way. Read the bottom *and* yourself at all times. That schizoid part also has to be thinking several steps ahead while being adaptable, all at the same time. In more than one scene I could tell the faggot's level of fear was getting dangerously high, so I had to move things forward to the climax before it all got out of hand.

And bottoms, you have shit to do too. First off, you've got to be *readable* if your schizo Top is going to have any chance to keep things fun. That means being in the moment and communicating where you are in terms of fear or arousal. Yeah, okay, maybe you can't make your dick hard or your pussy wet on command, but you can certainly control your moans, your begging, even the look in your eyes—an intoxicating mix of fear and trust.

After

After the scene it's time for aftercare, as in any scene. Fear-based mindfucks tend to need the most aftercare. Step one: dissipate the danger. If you were using a gun, it's time to put it away. If the fag Jew is still looking at a swastika, his brain is still pumping out adrenaline. Remove all danger to stop the flow of adrenaline, then wait for them to come down. Remember, we're talking fight-or-flight here. It's gonna take them some time to come down from it all. After that, it's time to discuss what happened—what worked, what didn't, what went through whose mind when. And, hey, it's never a bad idea to check in a day or two later as well.

> Now, if a mindfuck is done right you can have all of the danger with none of the actual risk; for example, fake gun equals lots of danger and no risk.

HANDLING DANGER

Now, if a mindfuck is done right you can have all of the danger with none of the actual risk; for example, fake gun equals lots of danger and no risk. But still, because mindfuck is such a powerful scene (because so much of it happens up in the head), there are some real and serious risks to keep in mind. The biggest risk of most mindfucks is that the bottom will freak out. Fortunately, I've never had a bottom do that on me—probably more out of luck than skill, though. Still, I've thought about what to do in such a situation. Here are my recommendations:

1. First, absolutely remove all dangers, real or fake.

2. Second, ask the bottom what he needs. Anything you say or do without asking this first is what the psycho killer would do. What do I mean? Well, you offer him a drink—he thinks, *That's what the psycho killer would do.* You offer to hold her until she calms down—she thinks, *That's what the psycho killer would do.* You suggest that it's probably not a good idea to leave right now because

they're all jacked up on adrenaline—and they think what? Yep, you guessed it: *That's what the psycho killer would do.* But asking the bottom what he needs is different, because psycho killers don't do that.

3. Third, have the bottom call someone he or she knows and trusts. Again, the psycho killer would never do that (witnesses only create complications); it also reconnects the bottom to the real world. They may not feel sure of the real world at first. Ideally, they'll be able to chat with their friend until the they're calm enough for some real aftercare—getting that drink, being held, even leaving.

There is one other potential danger, but just for Tops. I don't know how big this danger is, really. Based on my experience, if you do a lot of mindfuck and you do it well, people will fear you. Depending on your local community, this could mean fewer partners. The flip side, of course, is that your new reputation will do most of the work for you. Heck, some folks won't ever believe I'm *not* mindfucking them. Kinda hot, kinda sucks.

FUCKING QUESTIONS

Lastly, there are some basic questions both bottoms and Tops will want to ask before any mindfuck. Two key questions come before all the others.

1. *When you are masturbating while thinking about this fantasy, at what point do you come?* The mindfuck need go no further than that point.

2. *How real would be too real?* Rape is a common fantasy and a good scene for a mindfuck. But how real can it be before it stops feeling like a scene and starts feeling like a real rape?

Here are some other questions you might ask, based on the kind of mindfuck you have in mind:

Fear-Based

What's the fear? (Some more or less universal ones are death, severe nonerotic pain, abandonment, loneliness, disappointment, failure.)

How can it be simulated?

How can you set the stage?

What is the sub expecting? Play to it or off it?

Where do you want it to start? Where do you want it to end?

Fantasy-Based

What's my fantasy? What specifics are key to me?

What about it turns me on?

What is behind this fantasy?

Faith-Based

What do you want to accomplish?

How far are you willing to go?
What might go wrong?

FUCK YOU

Normally, if I were teaching this as a class, this is the point where I would take questions. Can't really do that in an essay, so I'll leave you with this kicker: I've lied to you six times in this essay. Not about the important stuff, but about me. Which parts are the lies? Think you know? Want to find out? Easy. Give me one hour—just *one* hour—with you, alone in a room. Deal?

Endnotes

1 As a gay man, I am not allowed to marry, I am not allowed to donate blood, but I *am* allowed to call other gay men "faggot," especially when they get off on verbal abuse, which is most of the men I play with.

RESOURCE GUIDE

Note: You can find a much more extensive version of this resource guide on the book's website, UltimateGuideToKink.com.

BOOKS

Becoming a Slave, by Jack Rinella (Chicago: Rinella Editorial Services, 2005).

The Compleat Slave: Creating and Living an Erotic Dominant/Submissive Lifestyle, by Jack Rinella (Los Angeles: Daedalus Publishing, 1992).

Different Loving: The World of Sexual Dominance and Submission, by Gloria Brame and William Brame (New York: Villard, 1996).

Family Jewels: A Guide to Male Genital Play and Torment, by Hardy Haberman (Eugene, OR: Greenery Press, 2001).

Leatherfolk: Radical Sex, People, Politics, edited by Mark Thompson (Los Angeles: Daedalus Publishing, 2004).

Leathersex: A Guide for the Curious Outsider and the Serious Player, by Joseph Bean (Los Angeles: Daedalus Publishing, 1994).

The Marketplace (3rd ed.), by Laura Antoniou (Cambridge, MA: Circlet Press, 2010).

The Master's Manual: A Handbook of Erotic Dominance, by Jack Rinella (Los Angeles: Daedalus Publishing, 1994).

Miss Abernathy's Concise Slave Training Manual, by Christina Abernathey (Eugene, OR: Greenery Press, 1996).

The Mistress Manual: The Good Girl's Guide to Female Dominance, by Mistress Lorelei (Eugene, OR: Greenery Press, 2000).

The New Bottoming Book, by Dossie Easton and Janet Hardy (Eugene, OR: Greenery Press, 2001).

The New Topping Book, by Dossie Easton and Janet Hardy (Eugene, OR: Greenery Press, 2003).

Partners in Power: Living in Kinky Relationships, by Jack Rinella (Eugene, OR: Greenery Press, 2003).

Sacred Kink: The Eightfold Paths of BDSM and Beyond, by Lee Harrington (Lulu.com, 2010).

Screw the Roses, Send Me the Thorns: The Romance and Sexual Sorcery of Sadomasochism, by Philip Miller and Molly Devon (Fairfield, CT: Mystic Rose Books, 1995).

The Seductive Art of Japanese Bondage, by Midori (Eugene, OR: Greenery Press, 2002).

Sensuous Magic: A Guide for Adventurous Couples, by Patrick Califia (Berkeley: Cleis Press, 2002).

Shibari You Can Use: Japanese Rope Bondage and Erotic Macramé, by Lee Harrington (Brooklyn, NY: Mystic Productions Press, 2007).

The Slave (3rd ed.), by Laura Antoniou (Cambridge, MA: Circlet Press, 2011).

SM 101: A Realistic Introduction, by Jay Wiseman (Eugene, OR: Greenery Press, 1998).

The Toybag Guide to Age Play, by Lee Harrington (Eugene, OR: Greenery Press, 2008).

The Toybag Guide to Clips and Clamps, by Jack Rinella (Eugene, OR: Greenery Press, 2004).

The Toybag Guide to Foot and Shoe Worship, by Midori (Eugene, OR: Greenery Press, 2004).

The Toybag Guide to Playing with Taboo, by Mollena Williams (Eugene, OR: Greenery Press, 2004).

Two Knotty Boys Showing You the Ropes: A Step-by-Step, Illustrated Guide for Tying Sensual and Decorative Rope Bondage, by Two Knotty Boys (San Francisco: Green Candy Press, 2006).

Urban Tantra: Sacred Sex for the Twenty-First Century, by Barbara Carrellas (Berkeley, CA: Celestial Arts/Ten Speed Press, 2007).

When Someone You Love Is Kinky, by Dossie Easton and Catherine A. Liszt (Eugene, OR: Greenery Press, 2000).

VIDEOS

Midori's Expert Guide to Sensual Bondage, directed by Tristan Taormino (Vivid-Ed, 2009).

Nina Hartley's Guide Series. Nina Hartley hosts and Ernest Greene directs this DVD series covering domination, submission, bondage sex, spanking, and more (Adam and Eve, 2002–2008).

Penny Flame's Expert Guide to Rough Sex, directed by Tristan Taormino (Vivid-Ed, 2009).

The S/M Arts Collection: The Pain Game & Tie Me Up, hosted by Cleo Dubois (Academy of S/M Arts, 2002).

The SM Tech Educational Series. DVDs with accompanying short books, covering topics like flogging, spanking, bondage, and CBT and featuring educators Lolita Wolf, Joseph Bean, and Scott Smith (Nazca Plains Corporation, thenazcaplainscorp.com).

NATIONAL ORGANIZATIONS

Carter-Johnson Library, leatherlibrary.org
Leather Archives & Museum, leatherarchives.org
Masters and slaves Together International (MAsT), mast.net
National Coalition for Sexual Freedom, ncsfreedom.org
National Leather Association-International, nla-i.com
Woodhull Sexual Freedom Alliance, woodhullalliance.org

REGIONAL ORGANIZATIONS

Note: Many of these organizations also hold annual events; see their websites for more information.

Adventures in Sexuality, Columbus, OH, adventuresinsexuality.org
Arizona Power Exchange, Phoenix, AZ, arizonapowerexchange.org
Black Rose, Washington, DC, br.org
The Center for Sex Positive Culture, Seattle, WA, sexpositiveculture.org
Charlotte Area Power Exchange (CAPEX), Charlotte, NC, capex.info
Chicago Hellfire Club, Chicago, IL, hellfire13.org
The Exiles, San Francisco, CA, theexiles.org
The Group With No Name, Austin, TX, gwnn.net
LA-RAWW, Los Angeles, CA, laraww.com
Lesbian Sex Mafia, New York, NY, lesbiansexmafia.org
LRA, Chicago, IL, lra-chicago.org
MOB, Boston, MA, mobnewengland.org

National Leather Association (has local chapters in Arkansas, Atlanta, Colorado, Columbus, Central Florida, Dallas, Houston, Indianapolis, Oklahoma City, Northern Nevada, and Philadelphia), nla-i.com
New England Leather Alliance, Boston, MA, nelaonline.org
Portland Leather Alliance, Portland, OR, portlandleather.org
Society of Janus, San Francisco, CA, soj.org
TES, New York, NY, tes.org

SELECT EVENTS

Beat Me in St. Louis, St. Louis, MO, beatmeinstl.com
Beyond Leather, Fort Lauderdale, FL, beyondleather.net
Beyond Vanilla, Dallas TX, beyondvanilla.org
Black Beat, Baltimore, MD, blackbeatinc.org
Desire, Palm Springs, CA, desireleatherwomen.com
Fetish Fair Fleamarket, Boston, MA, fetishfairfleamarket.com
Folsom Fringe, San Jose, CA, folsomfringe.com
Great Lakes Leather Alliance Weekend, Indianapolis, IN, greatlakesleather.org
International Ms. Leather, San Francisco, CA, imsl.org
International Mr. Leather, Chicago, IL, imrl.com
Kinkfest, Portland, OR, kinkfest.org
Kinky Kollege, Chicago, IL, kinkycollege.com
Leather Leadership Conference, leatherleader.org
Master/slave Conference, Washington, DC, masterslaveconference.org
South Plains Leatherfest, Dallas, TX, southplainsleatherfest.com

Southeast Leatherfest, Atlanta, GA, seleatherfest.com
Shibaricon, Chicago, IL, shibaricon.com
Thunder in the Mountains, Denver, CO, thunderinthemountains.com
Tribal Fire, Oklahoma City, OK, tribalfireokc.com
Twisted Tryst, various locations, twistedtryst.com

WEB RESOURCES

BDSM Event Page, thebdsmeventspage.com
FetLife, fetlife.com
Hanky Code, leathernjonline.com/hanky.htm
Kink Academy, kinkacademy.com
Kink Aware Professionals, https://ncsfreedom.org/resources/kink-aware-professionals-directory/kap-directory-homepage.html

ABOUT THE CONTRIBUTORS

LAURA ANTONIOU (lantoniou.com) is the author of the well-known *Marketplace* series of erotic novels, now being published by Circlet Press; they are all being converted to e-books as well. She has also edited the groundbreaking *Leatherwomen* anthologies and several other collections of fiction and nonfiction. Her first book, *The Catalyst*, now renamed *Cinema Erotica*, is now available as an e-book through Ravenous Romance; the fiction she has written under her gay male pseudonym, Christopher Morgan, is being released under her real name as well. She travels around the world leading workshops for the alt-sex community, ranging from gentle introductions to role playing to weekend-long intensives on BDSM protocols. Follow her at her website or find her on Facebook, Fetlife, and other online communities.

PATRICK CALIFIA (née Pat Califia, prior to a gender transition from female to male) has been writing about sex practically since this activity was invented. SRSLY. He is the author of a dozen or so nonfiction and fiction books that explore the issue of sexual variation, the parameters of gender, and confronting the repression and social control of pleasure. He currently lives with his cute boy (six years and counting) and three fluffy, vogueing, caption-worthy kittehs, and hopes to welcome an Empowered Femme of Color to the household once everybody has moved from California to Florida. Patrick is currently doing research on FTM sexuality and working on a sex manual to accompany publication of the questionnaire data. But if you see him at a party, please don't ask him how the new book is coming!

BARBARA CARRELLAS (barbaracarrellas.com) is the author of *Urban Tantra: Sacred Sex for the Twenty-First Century* and *Luxurious Loving: Tantric Inspirations for Passion and Pleasure*. She is the founder of Urban Tantra®, an approach to sacred sexuality that adapts and blends conscious sexuality practices from Tantra to BDSM, and the cofounder of Erotic Awakening, a pioneering series of workshops focusing on the physical, spiritual, and healing powers of sex. Barbara was named Best Tantric Sex Seminar Leader in New York City by *Time Out New York* for her Urban Tantra® workshops. Barbara delights in blurring the lines between sacred and profane, enlightened and perverted, mystical and scientific, pleasure and pain. Barbara's most recent endeavors are her Urban Tantra® Professional Training Program (which, in its first year, graduated participants from 12 countries) and her new book, *Ecstasy Is Necessary*, a practical guidebook for ecstatic explorers (Hay House, 2012). Barbara is a proud graduate of the Coney Island Sideshow School with a double major in fire eating and snake handling.

EDGE is an author, mentor, teacher, and hard-core player from Florida with 20 years of experience in the scene. As his name and online moniker would suggest, he enjoys a wide range of edge play activities, from breath control to weaponsex, though he also has a passion for stogie scenes, clean Japanese rope bondage, and prolonged, intimate inner thigh beatings.

FIFTHANGEL (fifthangel@artofbdsm.com) has spent many of his nonworking weekends traveling throughout North America teaching at BDSM events for the last 11 years. He has written two books, *The Finer Points of Pain and Pleasure*, a how-to guide for using pressure points in BDSM scenes, and *Your Pain, My Pleasure: Inside the Mind of a Sexual Sadist*, as well as many magazine articles and interviews. FifthAngel and his wife, Katie, live a power-balanced, monogamous marriage that is very much SM oriented. Edge players in all aspects of their lives, they enjoy vertical rock and ice climbing, blasting zombies at the gun range, and whitewater rafting. When not dangling by a rope off the side of a mountain, they are at home on their five-acre farm on the outskirts of Denver, where they care for a growing family of animals.

HARDY HABERMAN (dungeondiary.blogspot.com) has been an active member of the leather community since the late 1970s and a member of many BDSM/fetish organizations, including NLA-International and Discipline Corps. He is a founding member of Inquisition Dallas. He is a gay activist, filmmaker, author, and speaker on aspects of the SM/leather scene. He was awarded NLA-I's Man of the Year award in 1999 and the NLA-I Lifetime Achievement award in 2007. In 2010, he received the National Gay and Lesbian Task Force Leather Leadership Award. Since April 1995, he and his boy, Patrick, have been living together in Dallas with their Feline Mistress, Elvira, and troublemaker Jack-the-Cat.

LEE HARRINGTON (PassionAndSoul.com) is a passionate spiritual and erotic educator, gender explorer, eclectic artist, and published author and editor on human sexuality and spiritual experience. He's been traveling the globe (from Seattle to Sydney, Berlin to Boston), teaching or talking about sexuality, psychology, kink, faith, magic, and desire since 1995, and has no intention of stopping anytime soon. Along his journey, he has been a brainy academic, a female adult film performer (under his previous name, Bridgett Harrington), a world-class sexual adventurer, an outspoken philosopher, a longtime sexuality and spirituality blogger (since 1998), a spirit worker and priest, and an award-winning writer and artist. Overall, Lee is a nice guy with a disarmingly down-to-earth approach to the fact that we are each a beautifully complex ecosystem, and we deserve to examine the human experience from that lens.

His books include *Shibari You Can Use: Japanese Rope Bondage and Erotic Macramé*, *Sacred Kink: The Eightfold Paths of BDSM and Beyond*, *The Toybag Guide to Age Play*, and *Shed Skins: Journeying in Self-Portraits*. He has worked as an anthology editor on such projects as *Rope, Bondage, and Power* and *Spirit of Desire: Personal Explorations of Sacred Kink*, while contributing actively to other anthologies, magazines, blogs, and collaborations internationally. Check out the trouble Lee has been getting into, as well as his regular podcast, tour schedule, free essays, videos, and more on his website.

MIDORI (www.FHP-inc.com) is a renowned educator and writer on sexuality and SM. Dubbed "the supernova of kink" by Dan Savage, she emerged from the Sex Positive Movement in San Francisco in the early 1990s, soon becoming a much sought after international presenter on sexuality, personal fulfillment, and kinky adventures. Considered a pivotal figure in the leather and BDSM communities, she is also a critic, activist, and agent provocateur. Her reputation as an authority and leading expert on alternative pleasures stems not only from her unique and entertaining process of teaching concrete skills, but from her ability to deconstruct and distill complex matters of desire into surprisingly accessible lessons with eloquence and humanity. She is known for tackling challenging topics with fresh and relevant insights, using what she calls her "head–heart–hands" method for creating a space where people are allowed individual self-exploration.

Midori is fundamentally motivated by a desire to help people create authentic and intimate relationships while emphasizing self-actualization, shame reduction, acceptance, and justice. She is the author of *The Seductive Art of Japanese Bondage, Wild Side Sex: The Book of Kink,* and *Master Han's Daughter,* as well as numerous articles and columns. In 2001, she founded Rope Bondage Dojo©. She has trained many cadres and still leads many dojos each year. More recently, she formed ForteFemme, a unique women's dominance weekend training and empowerment intensive. Born and raised in Japan, she is now a resident of San Francisco, where she shares a home with her wonderful spouse and severely spoiled four-legged furry beings.

For more than 17 years **JACK RINELLA** (*leathermusings.blogspot.com*) has been writing about kinky sex. He is the author of *The Master's Manual, The Compleat Slave, Partners in Power, The Toybag Guide to Clips and Clamps, Becoming a Slave,* and *Philosophy in the Dungeon, The Magic of Sex & Spirit, The Dictionary of Scene-Friendly Terms,* and *More from the Master.* He has been active in the leather scene since 1983, is a founding member of MAsT-Chicago, a member of the Chicago Hellfire Club, and serves as a director on the board of the Leather Leadership Conference.

IGNACIO RIVERA, aka Papí Coxxx (ignaciorivera.com) identifies as a queer, gender-fluid, polyamorous, kinky, Black-Boricua. Ignacio is a descendant of colonized and uprooted Taíno and African slaves. Ignacio's people are from Borikén, also known as Puerto Rico. Ignacio, who prefers the gender-neutral pronoun "they," is a lecturer, activist, sex worker, sex educator, and performance artist who performs spoken-word, one-person shows and storytelling internationally. Their body of work focuses on gender and sexuality, specifically queer, trans, kink, and sexual liberation issues within a race/class dynamic. Their written work has appeared in *ColorLines, Ebony, Yellow Medicine Review,* and in three chapbooks: *Las Alas* (coauthored with Maceo Cabrera Estévez), *Ingridients,* and *Thoughts, Rants and What Some Might Call Poetry.* Ignacio is the recipient of a Marsha A. Gómez Cultural Heritage Award from LLEGÓ: The National Latina/o Lesbian, Gay, Bisexual, and Transgender Organization. They are the creator of Poly Patao Productions (P3), which is dedicated to producing sex-positive workshops, performance pieces, play parties, panel discussions, teach-ins, social/political groups, and educational opportunities that are specially geared toward queer women, transgender, multigender, genderqueer, gender-nonconforming, and gender-variant folks of color. Ignacio is also one of the founding board members of Queers for Economic Justice, a progressive nonprofit organization committed to promoting economic justice in a context of sexual and gender liberation.

FELICE SHAYS (brutalaffection.com) thrives where respect, sex, playing hard, laughter, safety, love, and talking shit all intersect. She's a sex and BDSM educator and coach who travels throughout the U.S. and Canada teaching at events, sex-positive stores, universities, conferences, and community organizations. Felice has appeared on British TV and in national and international print and digital media (including *Marie Claire* and *The Village Voice*). Her hands-on work with individuals, couples, and other partnership configurations ignites mighty, sexy self-discovery. Felice's decade's worth of events and venues include Good For Her, Black Rose, Pacific Friction, Dark Odyssey, Lesbian Sex Mafia, SheBop, KinkFest, Thunder in the Mountains, and many others.

Formerly a longtime sex educator at Babeland and one of the coproducers of New York's famous sex and BDSM play party, Submit, this Brooklyn femme currently lives in Portland, Oregon, where she is an ASL interpreter, a Queer Jewish event host, and a performance artist. Her one-ish woman shows include *Felice Brutality*, *Jew Hungry?*, *PsychoSemitic*, *The Temporary Flesh*, and *The Possibility of Response*, which have been produced at numerous theaters and festivals in New York, Boston, San Francisco, Toronto, Portland, and Baltimore. Her shows require her to hang—singing—from the ceiling and fist watermelons (somewhat akin to her life off the stage). Her essay is an excerpt from her first book, *Brutal Affection: Playing with Rough Sex*, which is coming soon, she promises.

SARAH SLOANE (SarahSloane.net) spends her time educating and writing about sexuality (both traditional and alternative), alternative relationships, and the lines of sex, gender, and politics. She has presented at some of the largest alt-sex events in the U.S. and overseas, as well as at sex-positive boutiques and to professional groups and universities. Her writing has been featured in various online publications, on her website, and in a few anthologies. You can find out more about her work and her upcoming events on her website.

MOLLENA (MO) WILLIAMS (mollena.com), "Delicate, Trembling Flower of Submission"©, is a New York City born and raised writer, leatherwoman, actress, BDSM educator, fat fetish model, and executive pervert. In the kink and leather communities, she identifies as a power slave who submits to only one. She is extremely honored to have served as International Ms. Leather 2010 and Ms. San Francisco Leather 2009. Mollena is a coalition partner and supporter of the National Coalition for Sexual Freedom and a former board associate for the Folsom Street Fair, and she was featured on the Folsom poster for 2010.

Active in the leather and BDSM communities since 1996,

she keeps it real all over North America and Europe, teaching on myriad BDSM, leather, and kinkcentric topics. She is deeply honored to have been nominated for the 21st Annual Pantheon of Leather's Woman of the Year Award and the Northern California Regional Award. She is a founding member of San Francisco's Crowded Fire Theater Company, and she writes a blog called *The Perverted Negress*. Mo is the author of *The Toybag Guide to Playing with Taboo* and coauthor, with Lee Harrington, of the forthcoming book *Playing Well with Others*. She has been featured in many interviews and has written dozens of articles, including "BDSM and Playing with Race," which appears in *Best Sex Writing 2010*.

LOLITA WOLF (leatheryenta.com) is a native New Yorker who discovered the BDSM scene back in the late 80s when "online" meant being on the phone sex lines. She is an activist who defends the sexual freedom of all consenting adults, spreads the word about BDSM, sex, and poly, and helps the community grow and flourish. Yet her goal remains to have fun. Lolita's many specialties include bondage, sensation and impact play of all sorts, poly relationships, and social skills. She has taught for organizations across the country, including TES, GMSMA, Black Rose, Living in Leather, South Plains Leatherfest, Thunder in the Mountains, Portland Kinkfest, Frolicon, Dark Odyssey, and many others, and she has presented seminars at Columbia, Yale, NYU, The New School, Bard, and Rutgers. Lolita is an emeritus board member of the Leather Leadership Conference and The Eulenspiegel Society (TES). She is a former Chair of Lesbian

Sex Mafia, an honorary member of GMSMA, and an associate member of New York boys of Leather. She is active with the National Coalition for Sexual Freedom and Leather Pride Night.

Lolita is the author of *Spanking* and *CBT in a Nutshell*. Her writing has appeared in *On Our Backs*, *Prometheus*, and *The Lust Chronicles*. Recently, she was featured in the *New York Times*'s "One in 8 Million" series. A six-year-old Princess who lies about her age, Lolita manages to stir up shit and get her own way (mostly). She is part of a far-ranging leather family and considers herself a versatile opportunist.

MADISON YOUNG (feministporn.net) is an international award-winning feminist porn star, director, gallerist, artist, and new mom. She has been called a "sex-positive Tasmanian devil." She has been directing and performing in erotic films for nearly a decade and has won great acclaim for her video line, Madison Young Productions, and her network of erotic websites, the Feminist Porn Network. Her films have screened at film festivals through out the States, Europe, and Australia. Young values sexual education in her work and has taught workshops and lectures and served as a panelist on the topics of sexuality, feminist pornography, and kink across the U.S., including at Yale University and UC Berkeley. She has recently finished a memoir, *Breathe: The Sexual Evolution of Madison Young*, based on her experiences in the adult industry, due out in spring 2012.

Madison has contributed writing to *Baby Remember My Name,* edited by Michelle Tea, *Rope Bondage and Power*

Exchange, edited by Lee Harrington, and *In-Soumises,* edited by Wendy Delorme. She has been featured in numerous documentaries including Virginie Despentes's *Mutantes: Feminisme PornoPunk* and has been featured on the Independent Film Channel, Spike TV, The History Channel, LOGO, MTV, and on HBO's *Real Sex.* When she isn't documenting hot sex on film, she is running her own nonprofit community art gallery in San Francisco, Femina Potens Art Gallery, which focuses on the expression of art, sex, and gender. Ms. Young resides in San Francisco with her partner and Dominant, James Mogul, and their daughter, Emma.

ABOUT THE ILLUSTRATOR

KATIE DIAMOND (katiediamond.com) is a radical queer comic artist and graphic designer. She graduated from the Maine College of Art with a Bachelor of Fine Arts in Illustration, where she got the nickname "Megaphone" because of her extensive community activism. She strongly believes in the direct crossover of art and politics, and uses this dogma in her everyday art practice. She has created many illustrations and cartoons about gender, sexuality, and sex education, and has designed a multitude of promotional materials for various local organizations. She is the publisher and editor of the queer feminist sex magazine *Salacious,* and her comic collaboration with queer performer Johnny Blazes is featured in the Lambda Literary Award–winning anthology *Gender Outlaws: The Next Generation.* She was named International Ms. Bootblack in April 2011.

ABOUT THE EDITOR

TRISTAN TAORMINO (tristantaormino.com and puckerup.com) is an award-winning author, columnist, editor, sex educator, and feminist pornographer. She is the author of seven books: *Secrets of Great G-Spot Orgasms and Female Ejaculation*, *The Big Book of Sex Toys*, *The Anal Sex Position Guide*, *Opening Up: A Guide to Creating and Sustaining Open Relationships*, *The Ultimate Guide to Anal Sex for Women*, *True Lust: Adventures in Sex, Porn and Perversion*, and *Down and Dirty Sex Secrets*. She has edited 23 anthologies, including her latest, *Take Me There: Trans and Genderqueer Erotica*, and was the founding series editor of 16 volumes of the Lambda Literary Award–winning anthology *Best Lesbian Erotica*. She runs Smart Ass Productions, and has directed and produced more than 20 adult films, from sex education to reality porn. She has written for a multitude of publications from *Yale Journal of Law and Feminism* to *Penthouse*, and is a former editor of *On Our Backs* and a former syndicated columnist for *The Village Voice*. She has appeared in hundreds of publications and on radio and television. She lectures at top colleges and universities and teaches sex and relationship workshops around the world. She lives with her partner and their dogs in upstate New York.

CPSIA information can be obtained
at www.ICGtesting.com
Printed in the USA
LVHW090316240522
719589LV00015B/860